DIE NAHRUNG
FOOD

Chemistry
Biochemistry
Microbiology
Technology
Nutrition

Edited by the
Central Institute of Nutrition
of the Academy of
Sciences of the GDR

Volume 32
1988
Number
9

Akademie-Verlag · Berlin

ISSN 0027-769X
Nahrung, Berlin 32 (1988) 9, 805–924

Instructions to Authors

1. Only papers which are valuable in content and which have not been published or submitted elsewhere will be accepted.

2. Manuscripts must be written in German or English, double-spaced on one side of the paper only.

3. Manuscripts should be submitted in the original (not as copies) to:
Editorial office "Die Nahrung — Food"
c/o Central Institute of Nutrition, Arthur-Scheunert-Allee 114—116, Bergholz-Rehbrücke, DDR-1505.
The receipt and acceptance of work will be confirmed in writing.

4. The institutes where the paper originates should be stated at the head of the manuscript. Next should follow its title and the name of its authors (with preceding initials).

5. The paper should begin with a summary (maximum 25 typed lines) which gives the content and conclusions of the work in concise and informative form. This should be presented so that it can be directly used or easily adapted for abstract journals. The addition of translations into Russian and English (or German) is desirable.

6. As far as possible, papers should be divided into:
   - Short introduction (present position of knowledge, statement of problems)
   - Materials and methods
   - Results and discussion (if necessary, divided into two parts).

7. The double presentation of results in both figures and tables should be avoided.

8. Graphs and structural formulas must be very accurately drawn and — as in the case of half-tone illustrations — of a quality suitable for reproduction. All legends should be typed together on a separate sheet of paper.

9. Tables should be appended to the manuscript on separate sheets.

10. Literature references should be specified at the end of the contribution as follows:
With books, under authors with initials, the title in the original language (Cyrillic transliterated), edition, page numbers (if necessary), publisher, place and year.
With edited books the editors should be named after the title: 'edited by ...'.
With journal papers, under all authors with initials, title of journal in the accepted abbreviation, volume number (underlined), year of publication (in brackets), issue number (if no continuous page numeration in the whole volume is given), page numbering. For example: Dam, T. G. J., R. E. Eshenbruch and D. J. Kitchen, Food Technol. New Zealand 6 (1982) 3, p. 22, 24, 26—29.

11. The nomenclature of chemical compounds and their written form should as far as possible conform to the IUPAC regulations.

12. Only SI units should be used.

13. At the end of the contribution the addresses of the authors (or only that of the corresponding author) should be given. From female authors we courteously request the forename in full.

14. The Editorial Board reserves the usual right to the editorial revising of the manuscript. However, major alterations will only be undertaken with the agreement of the authors.

15. The authors receive page proofs, in which only misprints and unavoidably necessary corrections should be considered.

16. Short communications (maximum 4 typed pages including tables and illustrations ready for reproduction) will be published more quickly (without summaries). The authors receive no sheets for correction, but there will be an editorial proof-reading.

17. Upon request up to 70 offprints of each paper will be supplied to the authors free of charge. Additional offprints may be ordered at cost price.

DIE NAHRUNG

FOOD

Founded by A. Scheunert and K. Täufel
Edited by the Central Institute of Nutrition of the Academy of Sciences of the GDR
(Director: Prof. Dr. habil. H. Schmandke)

mber 9
lume 32 · 1988

Akademie-Verlag · Berlin

'Die Nahrung — Food' publishes experimental results as original papers or as promptly issued short communications and state-of-the art reviews from the entire range of food and human nutrition. Therefore this journal is of interest to everyone working in this field — above all food chemists, technologists, and hygienists, nutritional physiologists and sociologists, physicians and microbiologists.

Bestellungen sind zu richten

- **in der DDR** an das Zeitungsvertriebsamt der Deutschen Post, Abt. Zentralvertrieb Berlin, Straße der Pariser Kommune 3—4, DDR-1004 Berlin, oder an den Akademie-Verlag Berlin, Leipziger Str. 3—4, DDR-1086 Berlin;
- **im sozialistischen Ausland** an eine Buchhandlung für fremdsprachige Literatur oder an den zuständigen Postzeitungsvertrieb;
- **in der BRD und in Berlin (West)** an eine Buchhandlung oder an die Auslieferungsstelle Kunst und Wissen, Erich Bieber oHG, Postfach 102844, D-7000 Stuttgart 10;
- **in den übrigen westeuropäischen Ländern** an eine Buchhandlung oder an die Auslieferungsstelle Kunst und Wissen, Erich Bieber GmbH, General Wille-Str. 4, CH-8002 Zürich;
- **im übrigen Ausland** an den Internationalen Buch- und Zeitschriftenhandel; den Buchexport, Volkseigener Außenhandelsbetrieb der Deutschen Demokratischen Republik, Postfach 160, DDR-7010 Leipzig; oder an den Akademie-Verlag Berlin, Leipziger Str. 3—4, DDR-1086 Berlin.

Orders can be sent

- **in the GDR** to the Zeitungsvertriebsamt der Deutschen Post, Abt. Zentralvertrieb Berlin, Straße der Pariser Kommune 3—4, DDR-1004 Berlin, or to the Akademie-Verlag Berlin, Leipziger Str. 3—4, DDR-1086 Berlin;
- **in the other socialist countries** to a book-shop for foreign literature or to the competent news distributing agency;
- **in the FRG and Berlin (West)** to a book-shop or to the wholesale distributing agency Kunst und Wissen, Erich Bieber oHG, Postfach 102844, D-7000 Stuttgart 10;
- **in the other Western European countries** to a book-shop or to the wholesale distributing agency Kunst und Wissen, Erich Bieber GmbH, General Wille-Str. 4, CH-8002 Zürich;
- **in other countries** to the international book- and journal-selling trade; to Buchexport, Volkseigener Außenhandelsbetrieb der DDR, Postfach 160, DDR-7010 Leipzig; or to the Akademie-Verlag Berlin, Leipziger Str. 3—4, DDR-1086 Berlin.

Zeitschrift „Die Nahrung — Food“
Herausgeber: Der Direktor des Zentralinstituts für Ernährung der Akademie der Wissenschaften der Deutschen Demokratischen Republik.
Verlag: Akademie-Verlag Berlin, Leipziger Str. 3—4, DDR-1086 Berlin;
Fernruf: 2236201 oder 2236229; Telex-Nr.: 114420; Bank: Staatsbank der DDR, Kto.-Nr.: 6836-26-20712.
Redaktion: Dr. Joachim Voigt (Chefredakteur), Dr. Ulrich Behnke.
Anschrift der Redaktion: Zentralinstitut für Ernährung der Akademie der Wissenschaften der DDR, Arthur-Scheunert-Allee 114—116, DDR-1505 Bergholz-Rehbrücke; Fernruf: Bergholz-Rehbrücke 8227.
Veröffentlicht unter der Lizenznummer 1287 des Presseamtes beim Vorsitzenden des Ministerrates der Deutschen Demokratischen Republik.
Gesamtherstellung: VEB Druckerei „Thomas Müntzer“, DDR-5820 Bad Langensalza.
Erscheinungsweise: Die Zeitschrift „Die Nahrung — Food“ erscheint jährlich in einem Band mit 10 Heften. Bezugspreis je Heft 27,— DM; Bandpreis 270,— DM zuzüglich Versandspesen. Der gültige Jahresbezugspreis für die DDR ist der Postzeitungsliste zu entnehmen.
Bestellnummer des Heftes: 1054/32/9.

AN (EDV) 64914 — AN (ZV) 111 800 012 8
01300

Die Nahrung 32 (1988) 9, 807—814

Hygiene-Institut Dessau (Direktor: OMR Dr. med. M. BAUER), Dessau, DDR

Untersuchungen zum Nickelgehalt von Lebensmitteln

G. RUICK

In 933 Lebensmitteln (Marktproben aus einem stark industrialisierten Gebiet der DDR) wird der Nickelgehalt mit Hilfe der Flammen-AAS und der Adsorptionsvoltammetrie bestimmt. Ein Vergleich der mit beiden Analysenverfahren erhaltenen Resultate zeigt, daß signifikante Abweichungen nicht auftreten. Die ermittelten Nickelgehalte stimmen gut mit vergleichbaren Werten aus der Literatur überein. Eine Abschätzung der alimentären wöchentlichen Nickelaufnahme auf der Grundlage der Angaben des statistischen Jahrbuches der DDR ergab einen Wert von 1,05 mg Ni pro Person.

Einleitung

Nickel wird zu den essentiellen Spurenelementen gerechnet. Über den Gehalt von Lebensmitteln an diesem Element liegen bisher aus der DDR nur wenige detaillierte Angaben vor. KRONEMANN u. a. [1] führten orientierende Untersuchungen über das Vorkommen von Nickel in pflanzlichen Lebensmitteln durch. ELLEN u. a. [2] bestimmten die Nickelkonzentration in Lebensmitteln aus den Niederlanden. Angaben über die Nickelgehalte einzelner Lebensmittel wurden auch aus verschiedenen anderen Ländern bekannt [2, 3]. Pflanzliche Lebensmittel zeigten höhere Konzentrationen an Nickel als tierische [4]. Besondere Bedeutung maß man den mit Tabakrauch inhalierten Nickelverbindungen bei [5]. SZADKOWSKI u. a. [6] ermittelten im Gesamtstromrauch einer Zigarette durchschnittlich 0,225 µg Ni. Weitere Kenntnisse über den Nickelgehalt von Lebensmitteln sind zur Abschätzung der Nickelaufnahme bzw. -belastung der Bevölkerung unbedingt erforderlich.

Ziel dieser Arbeit ist, den Gehalt an Nickel in möglichst vielen Lebensmitteln zu bestimmen, damit eine Abschätzung der Nickelversorgung der Bevölkerung über Lebensmittel möglich wird.

Analytik

Zur Bestimmung von Nickel im Spurenbereich wurden bisher verschiedene analytische Verfahren herangezogen. Mit Hilfe photometrischer Methoden [7—11] konnten Erfassungsgrenzen von 0,2 µg Ni/cm^3 erreicht werden. In der neueren Literatur wird die Atomabsorptionsspektralphotometrie (AAS) mit Flammen-Anregung oder mit flammenloser elektrothermaler Atomisierung häufig beschrieben. Mittels Flammen-AAS wurden Erfassungsgrenzen von 0,02 µg Ni/cm^3 [1, 2, 12, 13, 14], mittels flammenloser AAS von 20 pg erhalten [13, 15].

Für die Analytik von Schwermetallspuren haben sich polarographische und voltammetrische Verfahren als besonders leistungsfähig erwiesen, wobei man mit der Square-wave-Polarographie und der Differentiellen Pulse-Polarographie in Verbindung mit einem Anreicherungsschritt („Stripping-Verfahren") der flammenlosen AAS ähnliche Nachweisgrenzen erzielte [16—21].

Eigene Untersuchungen

Unter Berücksichtigung der analytischen Erfordernisse sowie der vorhandenen apparativen Voraussetzungen werden die Flammen-AAS und die Adsorptions-Voltammetrie zur Bestimmung von Nickel in Lebensmitteln eingesetzt. Die Entfernung der organischen Matrix ist der erste wichtige Schritt bei der Ermittlung der Nickelkonzentration in Lebensmitteln. Der trockenen Veraschung im Muffelofen bei 420 °C in Quarzschalen wird wegen des geringen Personalaufwandes hierbei der Vorzug gegeben. Veraschungshilfen werden nicht zugesetzt. Verluste an Nickel treten bei der trockenen Veraschung nicht auf, wie anhand von Wiederfindungsversuchen (Tab. 1) sowie mittels eines Vergleiches mit einer Naßveraschung ($HNO_3/HClO_4$) gezeigt werden konnte. Nach Trockenveraschung werden 95—98% der nach Naßveraschung erhaltenen Werte gefunden.

Die Nachweisgrenze der Flammen-AAS ist für die Nickelbestimmung in den meisten Lebensmitteln ausreichend, wenn man 5—10 g Lebensmittel der Veraschung zuführt. Die Asche wird mit 1 M HCl befeuchtet und vorsichtig auf dem Wasserbad zur Trockne gebracht und in 1 M HCl gelöst. Die Komplexierung des Nickels mit Ammonium-Pyrrolidindithiocarbamat und anschließende Extraktion in Methyl-isobutylketon [22] hat sich zur Minimierung möglicher Interferenzen und zur Anreicherung des Nickels gut bewährt. Die Messung erfolgt am AAS 1 des VEB Carl Zeiss Jena bei 232 nm in einer Luft-Acetylen-Flamme. Standardabweichung: 0,02 bei $n = 11$ u. $\bar{x} = 0{,}64$ mg/kg; Nachweisgrenze: 40 ng Ni/cm^3 Meßlösung.

Die von Pihlar u. a. [18] angegebene Arbeitsvorschrift wird für die vorhandenen Voraussetzungen so modifiziert, daß ein Aliquot der für die AAS gewonnenen Aufschlußlösung auch zur Adsorptionsvoltammetrie eingesetzt werden kann. Als Komplexbildner werden 50 µl einer 0,1 M Lösung von Dimethylglyoxim in Ethanol zu 10 ml Meßlösung zugesetzt. Als Grundelektrolyt dient 1 M NH_3/1 M NH_4Cl-Lösung (suprapur, Merck). Es wird in der Regel mit der Square-wave-Technik gearbeitet, lediglich bei sehr geringen Ni-Konzentrationen kommt die Differentielle Pulse-Technik zur Anwendung. Es werden die Ge-

Tabelle 1
Wiederfindungsraten für die Nickelbestimmung in Lebensmitteln nach Trockenveraschung
(Lebensmittel: Weizenmehl; Ni als $Ni(NO_3)_2$-Lösung zugegeben)

Zugabe [mg/kg]	gefunden [mg/kg]	Wiederfindungsrate [%]
0	0,63	—
0,07	0,68	95,2
0,10	0,72	96,7
0,20	0,84	99,5
0,50	1,12	99,3

Tabelle 2
Vergleiche der Nickelbestimmung in Lebensmitteln mittels Flammen-AAS und Adsorptionsvoltammetrie [mg/kg]

Lebensmittel	AAS	Ads.-Voltammetrie
Bockwurst	0,07	0,083
Leberwurst	0,07	0,068
Knoblauch-Rohwurst	0,037	0,032
Tomate	0,025	0,034
Paprika	0,037	0,021
Kartoffeln	0,056	0,056
Blumenkohl	0,050	0,047
Weißkohl	0,125	0,127
Äpfel	0,025	0,022
Stachelbeere	0,050	0,047

räte OH 104 der Fa. Radelkis, Budapest, oder PA 3 der Firma Laboratornije pristoje, Prag, benutzt. Als Meßelektrode dient eine hängende Quecksilbertropfelektrode (Kemula-Typ), als Gegenelektrode eine Ag/AgCl-Elektrode und als Hilfselektrode eine Pt-Blech-Elektrode. Das Adsorptionspotential wird auf —0,7 V eingestellt, das Peakpotential liegt bei —1,0 V. Die Nachweisgrenze liegt bei einer 2 min. Anreicherungszeit bei 5 ng/cm^3 Meßlösung für die Square-wave-Technik und bei 0,01 ng/cm^3 Meßlösung für die Differentielle Pulse-Technik. Relative Standardabweichung 10,2% bei $n = 10$; $\bar{x} = 0{,}047$ mg/kg.

Vergleichende Untersuchungen zur Nickelbestimmung in Lebensmitteln mit der Flammen-AAS und der Adsorptionsvoltammetrie werden an den verschiedensten Lebensmitteln durchgeführt (Tab. 2). Ein Vergleich der Ergebnisse mit Hilfe des t-Testes nach STUDENT [23] zeigt, daß die Abweichungen zwischen beiden angewendeten Bestimmungsmethoden im Bereich der zufälligen Fehler liegen ($n = 10$; $P = 0{,}95$; t-Wert nach Tabelle: 2,262; errechneter t-Wert: 0,191).

Ergebnisse

Den in Tab. 3 angeführten Ergebnissen liegen die Werte von 933 Analysen pflanzlicher und tierischer Lebensmittel zu Grunde. Die Standardabweichung sowie das Vertrauensintervall wurden nach [23] und [24] berechnet.

Die Lebensmittel sind Marktproben und wurden im Rahmen der öffentlichen Lebensmittelkontrolle in einem stark industrialisierten Gebiet der DDR entnommen. Sie wurden vor der Veraschung haushaltsmäßig gereinigt. Alle Angaben beziehen sich auf das Frischgewicht der Lebensmittel. Vergleicht man diese Daten mit den in der Literatur mitgeteilten Werten [1, 2], so lassen sich größere Unterschiede zu anderen europäischen Ländern nicht feststellen. Die teilweise sehr großen Vertrauensintervalle sind auf verschiedene Faktoren, z. B. die geographische Herkunft, zurückzuführen. Als reiche Nickellieferanten können Getreide, Kartoffeln und Gemüse gelten, ebenso viele häufig verzehrte tierische Lebensmittel; Milch, Obst und die meisten Getränke weisen nur sehr geringe Nickelgehalte auf. Schätzt man die wöchentliche Nickelzufuhr über Lebensmittel anhand der Angaben des statistischen Jahrbuches der DDR [25] ab, so erhält man einen Wert von 1,05 mg Ni/Woche und Person.

Tabelle 3
Nickelgehalte von Lebensmitteln

Lebensmittel	untersuchte Proben n	Mittelwert $\bar{x}$ [mg/kg]	Vertrauensintervall $\Delta\bar{x}$ ($P = 0{,}90$)	Standardabweichung s
Tierische Lebensmittel				
Frischfleisch				
Rindfleisch	9	0,034	± 0,019	0,03
Schweinefleisch	21	0,018	± 0,01	0,023
Hammelfleisch	2	0,015	–	–
Broilerfleisch	13	0,036	± 0,023	0,048
Wildschweinfleisch	6	0,099	± 0,054	0,067
Rehfleisch	7	0,385	± 0,56	0,774
Innereien				
Schweineniere	11	0,044	± 0,030	0,056
Wildschweinniere	5	0,245	± 0,152	0,160
Rehniere	7	0,153	± 0,039	0,054
Rinderleber	15	0,193	± 0,10	0,237
Schweineleber	9	0,275	± 0,14	0,237
Wildschweinleber	5	0,402	± 0,22	0,231
Rehleber	5	0,096	± 0,033	0,035
Fleischprodukte				
Schweinefl. i. eig. Saft	2	0,050	–	–
Jagdwurst	2	0,193	–	–
Bockwurst	6	0,115	± 0,039	0,048
Knoblauch-Rohwurst	4	0,099	± 0,126	0,120
Leberwurst	6	0,080	± 0,021	0,026
Geflügellebercreme	3	0,034	–	–
Eier				
Hühnerei	11	0,077	± 0,013	0,024
Eigelb	4	0,137	± 0,052	0,045
Eiklar	4	0,057	± 0,024	0,021
Milch u. -produkte				
Trinkvollmilch	12	< 0,003	–	–
Quark	3	< 0,01	–	–
Schmelzkäse	8	0,131	± 0,066	0,100
Butter	10	0,006	–	0,007
Frischfisch				
Hecht	2	0,026	–	–
Karpfen	2	0,033	–	–
Rotbarsch	1	< 0,005	–	–
Dorsch	2	0,02	–	–
Flunder	1	0,03	–	–
Plötze	2	0,006	–	–
Hering	2	0,033	–	–
Makrele	3	0,013	–	–
diverse Fischkonserven	53	0,056	± 0,008	0,036

Tabelle 3 (Fortsetzung)

Lebensmittel	untersuchte Proben n	Mittelwert $\bar{x}$ [mg/kg]	Vertrauensintervall $\Delta\bar{x}$ ($P = 0{,}90$)	Standardabweichung s
Pflanzliche Lebensmittel				
Frischgemüse				
Kartoffeln	20	0,067	± 0,014	0,037
Rotkohl	6	0,050	± 0,019	0,024
Weißkohl	10	0,069	± 0,017	0,030
Wirsingkohl	3	0,050	—	—
Blumenkohl	3	0,117	± 0,099	0,059
Rosenkohl	1	0,12	—	—
Grünkohl	3	0,138	—	—
Chinakohl	1	0,02	—	—
Chicoree	2	0,203	—	—
Bohnen (grün)	3	0,077	—	—
Porree	3	0,041	—	—
Kohlrüben	4	0,07	± 0,029	0,025
Rhabarber	3	0,05	—	—
Zwiebeln	4	0,049	± 0,030	0,026
Kohlrabi	6	0,06	± 0,035	0,043
Sellerie	1	0,13	—	—
Rote Beete	2	0,06	—	—
Möhren	7	0,028	± 0,027	0,038
Tomaten	12	0,023	± 0,020	0,039
Gurken	19	0,013	± 0,006	0,016
Gemüsekonserven				
Junge Brechbohnen	5	0,26	± 0,215	0,226
Erbsen	7	0,415	± 0,197	0,27
Tomatenmark	9	0,29	± 0,120	0,194
Tomatenketchup	5	0,216	± 0,015	0,016
Mischgemüse	3	0,125	—	—
Rote Beete	4	0,104	± 0,056	0,048
Weinsäuerkraut	2	0,070	—	—
Brot, Mehle, Getreideprodukte				
Roggen-Mischbrot	15	0,083	± 0,019	0,044
div. Spezialbrote (Landbrote, Schrotbrote)	12	0,143	± 0,038	0,075
Weißbrot	6	0,070	± 0,033	0,041
Weizenmehl	9	0,058	± 0,013	0,021
Roggenmehl	3	0,103	—	—
div. Teigwaren	10	0,093	± 0,012	0,022
Fertigsuppen				
Rindfleischsuppe m. Reis	2	0,315	—	—
Rindfleischsuppe m. Eierteigwaren	6	0,630	± 0,686	0,836
Voigtländ. Kartoffelsuppe	1	0,102	—	—
Kalbfleischsuppe	1	0,20	—	—
Kindernahrungen				
auf Gemüsebasis	27	0,065	± 0,011	0,035

Tabelle 3 (Fortsetzung)

Lebensmittel	untersuchte Proben *n*	Mittelwert $\bar{x}$ [mg/kg]	Vertrauensintervall $\Delta\bar{x}$ ($P = 0{,}90$)	Standardabweichung *s*
auf Obstbasis	15	0,092	± 0,029	0,065
Kinderzusatznahrung (Säfte)	11	0,056	± 0,010	0,020
Gewürze				
Pfeffer	7	0,678	± 0,148	0,203
Zimt	2	0,7	—	—
Paprika, scharf	2	1,75	—	—
Paprika, edelsüß	2	1,50	—	—
Senfkörner	6	1,57	± 1,09	1,33
Kümmel	3	2,75	—	—
Nelken	4	0,55	± 0,14	0,12
Koriander	3	1,7	—	—
Lorbeerlaub	1	0,8	—	—
Einlegegewürz	2	1,55	—	—
Petersilie, getrockn.	2	1,41	—	—
Senf	3	0,156	—	—
Zucker	4	< 0,005	—	—
Frischobst				
Äpfel	9	0,015	± 0,009	0,016
Birnen	5	0,041	± 0,028	0,023
Pflaumen	3	0,093	—	—
Pfirsiche	3	0,215	—	—
Johannisbeeren, rot	2	0,05	—	—
Orangen	3	0,015	—	—
Zitronen	2	0,22	—	—
Grapefruit	1	0,05	—	—
Obstkonserven				
Erdbeeren	6	0,084	± 0,086	0,106
Apfelmus	6	0,016	± 0,022	0,028
Mischobst	2	0,275	—	—
Mandarinen	4	0,127	± 0,015	0,012
div. Marmeladen	17	0,105	± 0,019	0,047
Honig	12	0,009	± 0,007	0,015
Süßmoste und alkoholfreie Getränke				
Apfelsaft	29	0,088	± 0,035	0,114
Schwarzer Johannisbeer-Süßmost	10	0,067	± 0,025	0,044
Sauerkirsch-Süßmost	7	0,072	± 0,060	0,082
Rhabarber-Süßmost	12	0,077	± 0,040	0,078
Apfel-Orange-Nektar	7	0,033	± 0,031	0,043
Rhabarber-Nektar mit Orange	7	0,109	± 0,050	0,069
Birne-Orange-Nektar	7	0,033	± 0,021	0,030
Pflaumen-Orange-Nektar	5	0,024	± 0,010	0,011
div. Limonaden	50	< 0,002	—	—
div. Cola-Getränke	51	0,005	± 0,001	0,008

Tabelle 3 (Fortsetzung)

Lebensmittel	untersuchte Proben n	Mittelwert $\bar{x}$ [mg/kg]	Vertrauensintervall $\Delta\bar{x}$ ($P = 0,90$)	Standardabweichung s
Selterswasser	62	< 0,002	—	—
Bitter Tonic	3	< 0,002	—	—
Bier	6	0,021	± 0,017	0,020
Wein				
div. Weißweine	43	0,072	± 0,017	0,068
div. Rotweine	6	0,043	± 0,025	0,031
Spirituosen				
Korn	4	0,004	± 0,004	0,004
div. Weinbrände	4	0,030	± 0,016	0,014
Pflanzliche Fette				
Salatöl	3	0,008	—	—
Margarine	5	0,0592	± 0,055	0,075

Dieses Resultat ist in guter Übereinstimmung mit der von MYRON [26] und SCHROEDER [27] mitgeteilten Nickelaufnahme von 165 µg bzw. 300—600 µg pro Tag und Person. Eine Nickel-Unterversorgung ist nach diesen Ergebnissen für die DDR-Bevölkerung nicht zu befürchten, wenn man den auf 100 µg geschätzten täglichen Nickelbedarf [28] mit der tatsächlich aufgenommenen Nickelmenge vergleicht.

Summary

G. RUICK: Nickel content of foodstuffs

Using adsorption-voltammetry and atomic absorption spectrometry, the author determined the nickel contents in 933 foodstuff-samples (market samples from a highly industrialized region of the GDR). The values found agreed well with data from the literature. The weekly nickel intake via foodstuffs is about 1,05 mg per person.

Резюме

Г. РУИКК: Исследования содержания никеля в пищевых продуктах

В 933 пищевых продуктах (товарные пробы из сильно индустриализированной области ГДР) с помощью пламенной атомно-адсобционной спектроскопии и адсорбционной вольтаметрии определялось содержание никеля. Сравнение полученных этими двумя методами результатов показывает, что достоверных отклонений не наблюдается. Полученные данные содержания никеля хорошо совпадают со сравнимыми данными из литературы. Оценка еженедельного поступления никеля с пищей на основе данных статистического ежегодника ГДР выявило значение 1,05 мг никеля на человека.

Literatur

[1] KRONEMANN, H., M. ANKE, S. THOMAS und E. RIEDEL, 3. Spurenelement-Symposium, S. 221—228. Jena 1980.

[2] ELLEN, G., G. VAN DEN BOSCH-TIBBESMA und F. F. DOUMA, Z. Lebensm.-Unters. u. -Forsch. **166** (1978) 145—147.
[3] SCHLETTWEIN-GSELL, D., und S. MOMMSEN-STRAUB, Intern. Z. Vit. u. Ernähr.-Forsch. **41** (1971) 429.
[4] ANKE, M., M. GRÜN, B. GROPPEL und H. KRONEMANN, Zbl. Pharmazie **121** (1982) 474—489.
[5] WEHNER, A. P., R. H. BUSCH, R. J. OLSON und D. K. CRAIG, Amer. Ind. Hyg. Ass. J. (1975) 801—810.
[6] SZADKOWSKI, D., H. SCHULTZE, K.-H. SCHOLLER und G. LEHNERT, Arch. Hyg. Bakt. **153** (1969) 1—8.
[7] NIELSCH, W., Analyt. Chem. **150** (1956) 114.
[8] FRIES, J., Spurenanalyse — erprobte photometrische Methoden. E. Merck-KG, Darmstadt.
[9] EZEKAALO, M., Anal. Chim. Acta **62** (1972) 220.
[10] TAYLOR, C. G., Analyst **81** (1956) 369.
[11] KOCH, O. G., und G. A. KOCH-DEDIC, Handbuch der Spurenanalyse Bd. 2, S. 879. Springer-Verlag, Berlin—Heidelberg—New York 1974.
[12] WELZ, B., Atomabsorptionsspektroskopie. Verlag Chemie, Weinheim/Bergstraße 1975.
[13] DITTRICH, K., Atomabsorptionsspektroskopie. Akademie-Verlag, Berlin 1982.
[14] PRICE, W. J., J. T. H. ROOS und A. F. CLAY, Analyst **95** (1970) 760.
[15] JIN LONG-ZHU und NI ZHE-MING, Z. anal. Chem. **321** (1985) 72—76.
[16] GEISSLER, M., und G. KUHNHARDT, Square-wave-Polarographie. VEB Deutscher Verlag für Grundstoffindustrie, Leipzig 1970.
[17] WEINZIERL, J., und F. UMLAND, Z. anal. Chem. **312** (1982) 608—610.
[18] PIHLAR, B., P. VALENTA und H. W. NÜRNBERG, Z. anal. Chem. **307** (1981) 337—346.
[19] UTO, M., Y. HOH und M. SUGAWARA, Z. anal. Chem. **321** (1985) 68—71.
[20] BRAUN, H., und M. METZGER, Z. anal. Chem. **318** (1984) 321—326.
[21] NAVRES, H.-D., P. VALENTA und H. W. NÜRNBERG, Z. anal. Chem. **317** (1984) 484—485.
[22] WOGGON, H., and D. JEHLE, Nahrung **20** (1980) 95—98.
[23] ECKSCHLAGER, K., Fehler bei chemischen Analysen. Akademische Verlagsgesellschaft Geest und Portig K.-G., Leipzig 1964.
[24] DOERFFEL, K., Statistik in der analytischen Chemie, VEB Deutscher Verlag für Grundstoffindustrie, Leipzig 1984.
[25] Statistisches Jahrbuch der DDR 1984, Staatsverlag der DDR, Berlin 1984.
[26] MYRON, B., J. Clin. Nutr. **31** (1978) 527; zit. bei [1].
[27] SCHROEDER, H. A., J. Chron. Dis. **15** (1962) 51.
[28] PRASAD, A. S., Trace Elements and Iron in Human Metabolism. Plenum Medical Book Comp., New York und London 1978.

Dr. rer. nat. G. RUICK, Hygiene-Institut Dessau,
Am Tivoli 1, Dessau, DDR-4500

Eingegangen 9. 4. 1987
nach Revision 21. 9. 1987

Die Nahrung **32** (1988) 9, 815—821

National Institute of Food Hygiene and Nutrition, Budapest, and
Vegetable Oil and Detergent Research Institute, Budapest, Hungary

Effect of interesterified dietary fat mixtures on various lipid indices and liver metal content of rats in fat-metabolism disturbance

Á. J. N. Zsinka, J. Perédi, K. Lindner-Szotyori and Gy. Biró

Adult male and female Wistar rats were fed isoenergetically for a 6 week period with a lipogenic diet containing a 20% fat mixture which caused fat-metabolism disturbance. One group consumed the mixture of sunflower oil and lard in a ratio of 0.91 P/S, the other group the interesterified form of the same mixture. The linoleic acid content of the mixtures was 0.4%. The fat mixture of the third group's diet was adjusted with soya oil to a linoleic-acid content of 0.8%. The results were compared to the control data obtained in rats fed with a normal diet. The changes in various lipid indices of the serum and the liver and the levels of some metals in the liver were analysed. It was found that

— in comparison to the control on the effect of the lipogenic diet the total lipid and cholesterol contents of the serum increased significantly in all groups (a significantly higher value being observed for the females than for the males) whereas the HDL-C content decreased. As to the effect of the fat mixtures there were no considerable difference;
— in the liver of the females a similar trend of high lipid values was observed with the consumption of the different fat mixtures; in the liver of males the interesterified fat mixture and the fat mixture with a higher linoleic acid content caused a significantly higher total lipid, triglyceride, and total cholesterol accumulation than the non-interesterified mixture;
— the iron content of the liver decreased in the males of all three groups, but more significantly with interesterification and increasing the linoleic-acid content of the diet, while in the females the zinc content of the liver decreased,
— our experimental model of the fat-metabolism disturbance seems to be suitable for the determination of the effects of slight dietary changes i.e. for the study of changes in food technology.

It has been found in our former studies that feeding a lipogenic diet with 20% fats which cause fat-metabolism disturbances, the diets influenced differently the lipid content of the serum and liver [4—6]. According to our assumptions based on these results besides, the effect of differences between the compositions of fats and fat mixtures, various aspects of the influences of food technological changes or of slight variations in the fatty-acid composition can be reasonably cleared during the development of the fat-metabolism disturbances. Consequently, in the present experiments we investigated wether technological changes, such as the interesterification of the fat mixture (i.e. the change in the structure of triglycerides) or a slight alteration in the composition, such as the increase of only one of the fatty acids, the linoleic-acid content, in the fat mixture could cause any change in the lipid indices and in the various metal content in the liver.

Materials and methods

20—20 adult male and female Wistar rats of (215 ± 8) g (OÉTI — National Institute of Food Hygiene and Nutrition, Budapest) were fed isoenergetically with a lipogenic diet for six weeks (the composition of the diet

Table 1
Composition of experimental diets

Group	I	II	III	IV
Diet	LATI normal	Synthetic lipogen with		
		65% lard + 35% sunflower oil mixture	65% lard + 35% sunflower oil mixture interesterified	65% lard + 25% sunflower oil mixture 10% soya oil
Fat [%]	5	20	20	20
P/S*	—	0,91	0,91	0,88
Linoleic acid [%]	—	0,4	0,4	0,8

* Polyunsaturated/saturated fatty acid ratio

has been published former [4]). This feed contained 20% fats. The control group was given a normal diet (LATI). The experimental groups are given in Table 1.

The fat mixture were composed in the way to approach the optimal value of P/S = 1.

The fatty acid composition of the fats was measured by gas chromatography and gave similar results to the calculated composition.

Interesterification of the fat mixture. The mixture of lard and sunflower oil was interesterified using the so called "non-directed" method [9] as follows: The mixture of 65% dietary lard and of 35% refined sunflower oil was agitated for 1 h at 90 °C in the presence of sodium methylate as catalyst, then the catalyst was inactivated, acetic acid added and washed with distilled water. Finally the water was removed with sodium sulphate. As the effect of a "random interesterification", the melting point of the mixture decreased, its melting range became wider. The amount of the liquid components increased at room temperature.

The feeding period, the mean food intake, and body mass of the rats were monitored. After a six weeks' feeding period blood was taken from their abdominal aorta and the organ weights (liver, heart, kidney, spleen) were measured. Relative organ weights for 100 g body mass were calculated. From the serum and from the liver (extracted according to the method of FOLCH et al. [1], the amount of total lipid was determined according to ZÖLLNER et al. [12], the triglyceride content by enzymatic BOEHRINGER test, the total cholesterol and the precipitated HDL-C level [7] by the enzymatic GÖDECKE test. The iron, copper and zinc content in the liver was evaluated by the gaschromatographical method of GERGELY et al. [3]. After the calculation of group means and SD, the significance of deviation was calculated by variance analysis [11]. The livers were prepared for histological examination (haematoxylin-eosine and fat-dying).

Results

Data on diet and energy intake of the groups are presented in Table 2. The energy-consumption means of the various groups did not show significant differences. The energy intake for 100 g body mass was slightly higher for female rats. Table 3 displays the data on body-mass gains. In the experimental and the control group the bodymass gain of female rats was significantly lower, in spite of the slightly higher energy intake, than that of males. As an effect of lipogenic diet, a by 20—40% increased body weight could be observed in the males which was not observed in the female rats.

Change in the relative organ masses could be seen only in the liver. The relative mass of the liver and the different metal-content values are given in Table 4. The lipogenic diet caused a significant increase in the relative liver mass in all experimental groups. No significant difference was observed among effects of various fats. The control metal values of the liver of males and females were similar. As an effect of the lipogenic diet, a more significant decreasing trend could be found for male rats in the iron content of the liver, compared to females, where the zinc content was lower than for males. In males, the group III compared

Table 2
Diet and energy intake of rats

Group	I	II	III	IV
	Males			
Diet intake				
— [g/100 g body mass]	6.2	5.6	5.6	5.5
— [Joule/100 g body mass]	97	98.3	98	96
	Females			
Diet intake				
— [g/100 g body mass]	7.5	6.6	6.7	6.7
— [Joule/100 g body mass]	118	115	117	117

Table 3
Body mass gain (average) [g/6 weeks]

Group	Males	Females
I	74 ± 6	40 ± 4
II	93 ± 8[a]	46 ± 4.5
III	108 + 9.7[a]	39 ± 3.8
IV	118[a]	36 ± 3.2

a = I—II, III, IV; $p < 0.05$

Table 4
Relative liver mass and Fe, Cu, Zn content of liver

Group	Males				Females			
	I	II	III	IV	I	II	III	IV
Relative liver mass [g/100 g body-mass]	2,21 ± 0,14	4,29[a] ± 0,33	4,4[a] ± 0,31	4,24[a] ± 0,41	2,38 ± 0,13	4,05[a] ± 0,35	4,24[a] ± 0,26	4,28[a] ± 0,49
Fe [µg/g liver]	161,11 ± 28,91	99,52[a] ± 23,05	73,78[ab] ± 18,83	81,34[ab] ± 14,68	154,83 ± 91,39	137,7 ± 46,55	143,25 ± 48,46	131,17 ± 41,83
Cu [µg/g liver]	3,68 ± 0,59	3,18 ± 0,66	2,79[a] ± 0,66	3,25 ± 0,78	3,58 ± 1,49	2,88 ± 1,4	2,74 ± 0,93	3,39 ± 1,03
Zn [µg/g liver]	43,26 ± 15,47	30,45[a] ± 5,4	41,03 ± 19,76	35,63 ± 16,61	30,15 ± 8,16	22,48[a] ± 6,59	21,97[a] ± 5,1	25,53 ± 5,51

a = I—II, III, IV; $p < 0,01$
b = II—III, IV; $p < 0,02$

Table 5
Serum lipid levels

Group	I	II	III	IV
	Males			
Total lipid	4.83	9.9[a]	11.3[a]	10.1[a]
[g/l]	± 0.93	± 2.7	± 2.3	± 2.0
Triglyceride	0.62	0.38[a]	0.53	0.53
[mmol/l]	± 0.25	± 0.15	± 0.27	± 0.43
Total cholesterol	1.62	3.42[a]	4.2[a]	3.7[a]
[mmol/l]	± 0.52	± 0.88	± 0.77	± 1.22
HDL-C	1.0	0.97	0.81	0.75
[mmol/l]	± 0.2	± 0.32	± 0.34	± 0.34
Total chol./HDL-C	1.62	3.88[a]	5.18[a]	4.9[a]
	Females			
Total lipid	3.24	20.6[a]	22.1[a]	23.2[a]
[g/l]	± 0.39	± 7.9	± 7.43	± 5.02
Triglyceride	0.79	0.39[a]	0.35[a]	0.33[a]
[mmol/l]	± 0.45	± 0.14	± 0.16	± 0.1
Total cholesterol	1.82	18.2[a]	21.4[a]	21.7[a]
[mmol/l]	± 0.25	± 8.8	± 7.8	± 7.8
HDL-C	1.16	± 0.6[a]	± 0.73[a]	± 0.54[a]
[mmol/l]	± 0.07	± 0.35	± 0.31	± 0.42
Total chol./HDL-C	1.54	30.3[a]	29.3[a]	40.1[a]

a = I—II, III, IV; $p < 0.05$

Table 6
Liver lipid contents

Group	I	II	III	IV
	Males			
Total lipid	85.8	372[a]	442[ab]	450[ab]
[mg/g]	± 17.8	± 48	± 77	± 48
Triglyceride	29.4	94.6[a]	136[ab]	147[ab]
[mg/g]	± 9.5	± 32	± 40	± 43
Total cholesterol	7.3	108[a]	134[ab]	124[ab]
[mg/g]	± 1.9	± 8.6	± 8.7	± 10.4
	Females			
Total lipid	75.5	387[a]	418[a]	408[a]
[mg/g]	± 17	± 38	± 41	± 65
Triglyceride	43.9	136[a]	110[a]	104[a]
[mg/g]	± 17	± 35	± 30	± 32
Total cholesterol	5.9	116[a]	132[a]	127[a]
[mg/g]	± 1.5	± 10.1	± 10.3	± 16.5

a = I—II, III, IV; $p < 0.05$
b = II—III, IV; $p < 0.05$

to group II — fed with fat of the same composition but in an interesterified form — and the group IV (having consumed more linoleic acid) showed lower iron levels in the liver as well. In female rats, no significant differences could be observed.

Lipid indices of the serum are summarized in Table 5. As an effect of lipogenic diet, different results were found for males and for females. In male rats, compared to the control group, the total lipid and total cholesterol content increased significantly but to a much smaller degree as in female rats, where a very high total lipid and total cholesterol and a reduced HDL-C content could be observed. As to the effect of fats no significant differences were observed. The triglyceride level decreased significantly in comparison to the control in female rats in all cases, and in males as an effect of the diet II.

The lipid indices of the liver can be seen in Table 6. Compared to the control values, the lipogenic diet caused increases of similar order; in the females no significant difference was observed as an effect of different fats, but in males, a higher accumulation of total lipid, triglyceride and total cholesterol was caused by the interesterified fat mixture compared to the non-treated one. Similar changes were caused by the fat mixture containing soy oil, as well.

In all experimental groups according to histological results fatty degeneration of liver cells was found exhibiting individual differences represented in the form of focal great-drops or diffuse small-drops. The connective tissue trabeculae became wider and many inflamed elements could be detected (leucocytes, lymphoid cells, monocytic, histocytic infiltration and connective tissue mobilisation were observed). All these lesions can be regarded as a secondary inflammation symptome associated with the parenchymatous (fatty) degeneration, i.e. the "alimentary steatosis" has appeared.

Conclusions

Changes in accordance with our former results [4—6] were observed under experimental conditions as the effect of our lipogenic diet: The lipid level of the serum and of the liver increased significantly compared to the control values. The sexual differences were represented very clearly: In females, the serum total lipid and total cholesterol level were significantly higher, while the triglyceride content was lower than in males, whereas the body-mass gain of males was significantly higher than in female rats. The lipid accumulation of the liver showed a similar trend, but in the female rats with lower values. Based on these findings it can be suggested that the fat mobilisation in females was much more intensive than in males. The degree of fatty tissue degradation was not investigated but the increased serum lipid transport of the females and the liver lipid accumulation besides their lower body-mass gain lead to the above conclusion. A further study of this problem can be carried out with the observation of fat excretion, and mainly of fat-mobilization time, that are to be cleared.

As an effect of the interesterification of mixed lard and sunflower oil, thc amount of triglycerides "C_{54}" (fatty acid containing 3×18 C atoms) increased and the triglycerides "C_{52}" decreased. Fatty acids in the normal lard do not follow the "random" distribution obtained by probability calculation. In our former experiment with a mixture of lard and soya oil, the fatty-acid composition evaluated by gas-chromatográphy approached the random distribution of the probability calculations [10]. According to the results of our present experiments, the amount of triglycerides containing three unsaturated and also the three saturated fatty acids increased as an effect of interesterification. Nevertheless, the interesterification of the fat mixture changed the biological effect: In male rats the liver lipid level increased. It can be presumed, that the interesterification of sunflower oil caused biologically unfavourably positioned fatty-acid bindings in the triglyceride structure. For this reason, the modification of the interesterification technology is planned. The liver lipid content increase was observed in male rats due to fat mixtures with linoleic acid content. These results indicate a more intensive sensitivity of males for fat-metabolism disturbances, as well.

The relations between the fat content of the diet and the different metal levels of the liver are not cleared yet. With the development of fat-metabolism disturbance the iron content of the liver decreased being in negative correlation with the total lipid and triglyceride content of the liver, and this could be observed only in male rats. It should be cleared, whether in the differences between sexes the hormon regulation or the differences in fat metabolism (lipid peroxidation) were involved. The results of histological examinations of the liver in the experimental groups fed with the lipogenic diet, show — similarly to changes in the lipid indices — the development of a fatty liver, the "alimentary steatosis" of various degrees.

It can be concluded from the results that our model for fat-metabolism disturbance induced by the lipogenic diet reacts sensitively to smaller differences as well, i.e. it can be well applied to control the changes of various factors of the diet.

Zusammenfassung

Á. J. N. Zsinka, J. Perédi, K. Lindner-Szotyori und Gy. Biró: Einfluß von umgeesterten Diät-Fettmischungen auf verschiedene Lipid-Indices und den Metallgehalt der Leber von Ratten mit gestörtem Fettstoffwechsel

Erwachsene männliche und weibliche Wistar-Ratten werden isoenergetisch für 6 Wochen mit einer lipogenen Diät gefüttert, die 20% einer Fettmischung enthält und eine Störung des Fettstoffwechsels hervorruft. Eine Gruppe erhält eine Mischung von Sonnenblumenöl und Schmalz (P/S = 0,91), die andere die umgeesterte Form der gleichen Mischung. Der Linolensäuregehalt der Mischungen beträgt 0,4%. Der Fettgehalt der dritten Gruppe ist mit Sojaöl auf einen Linolensäuregehalt von 0,8% eingestellt. Die Ergebnisse werden mit Kontrolldaten verglichen, die an Ratten mit normalem Futter erhalten werden. Die Veränderungen der verschiedenen Lipid-Indices des Serums und der Leber und die Gehalte einiger Metalle in der Leber werden ermittelt.

Es wird festgestellt, daß

- im Vergleich zur Kontrolle durch den Einfluß der lipogenen Diät der Gehalt an Gesamtlipiden und an Cholesterol im Serum in allen Gruppen signifikant erhöht wird (bei den Weibchen signifikant höher als bei den Männchen), während der Gehalt an HDL-C abnimmt. Zwischen den Fettmischungen bestehen keine signifikanten Differenzen;
- in den Lebern der Weibchen beim Verzehr der verschiedenen Fettmischungen ein ähnlicher Trend hoher Lipidwerte zu beobachten ist; in den Lebern der Männchen verursacht die umgeesterte Fettmischung und diejenige mit einem höheren Gehalt an Linolensäure eine signifikant höhere Anreicherung an Gesamtlipiden, Triglyceriden und Gesamtcholesterol im Vergleich zur nicht umgeesterten Fettmischung;
- der Gehalt an Eisen in der Leber der Männchen in allen drei Gruppen abnimmt, jedoch stärker signifikant bei Interesterifizierung und Erhöhung des Linolensäuregehaltes, während bei den Weibchen der Zinkgehalt der Leber abnimmt;
- unser experimentelles Modell der Fettstoffwechsel-Störung für die Ermittlung des Einflusses schwacher diätetischer Veränderungen, d. h. für das Studium lebensmitteltechnologischer Veränderungen, geeignet zu sein scheint.

Резюме

А. Й. Н. Жинка, Й. Переди, К. Линднер-Сотъори и Дъ. Биро: Влияние переэтерифицированных диететических жировых смесей на различные липидные показатели и содержание металла в печени крыс с нарушенным жировым обменом

Взрослые самки и самцы крыс линии Вистар 6 недель кормлились изоэнергетической липогенной диетой, которая содержала 20% жира и вызывала нарушение липидного обмена. Одна группа получила смесь подсолнечного масла и смалца (P/S = 0,91), другая переэстерифицированную форму этой же смеси. Содержание линоленовой кислоты смесей равнялось 0,4%. Содержание жира у третей группы с помощью соевого масла доводилось до содержания линоленовой кислоты 0,8%. Результаты сравнивались с контрольными данными, полученными у крыс с нормальной диетой. Изучались изменения различных липидных показателей сыворотки крови и печени и содержание некоторых металлов в печени.

Результаты показывают, что

— по сравнению с контролем под влиянием липогенной диеты достоверно увеличивается содержание общих липидов и холестерола в сыворотке крови всех групп (у самок достоверно больше чем у самцов), в то время как содержание HDL-холестерина уменьшается. Между жировыми смесями достоверной разницы не обнаруживолась;
— в печени самок при потреблении различных смесей жира наблюдается аналогичный тренд к высоким липидным показателям; в печени самцов жировая смесь с переэтерифицированными жирами и смесь с более высоким содержанием линоленовой кислоты приводят к достоверному увеличению накопления общих липидов, триглицеридов и общего холестерола по сравнению с непереэтерифицированной смесью;
— содержание железа в печени самцов всех трех групп уменьшается, однако достоверно более сильно при переэтерификации и увеличении содержания линоле́новой кислоты, в то время как у самок уменьшается содержание цинка в печени;
— наша экспериментальная модель нарушения жирового обмена годится, по-видимому, для исследования влияния слабых диететических изменений, т.е. для изучения технологических изменений пищевых продуктов.

References

[1] Folch, J., M. Lees and S. G. H. Stanley, J. biol. Chem. **235**, 2595—2598 (1957).
[2] Friedewald, H., Clin. Chem. **18**, 499—452 (1972).
[3] Gergely, A., and K. Lindner-Szotyori, Elelmiszerv. Közl. **22**, 212—219 (1976).
[4] J. N. Zsinka, Á., V. Földes and J. Perédi, Acta aliment. **17**, 43—51 (1988).
[5] J. N. Zsinka, Á., V. Földes, A. Gere, J. Szépvölgyi, J. Perédi and T. Thuróczy-Thiermayer, Acta aliment. (1988, at press).
[6] J. N. Zsinka, Á., V. Földes, A. Gere, J. Perédi and T. Thuróczy-Thiermayer, (1988, at press).
[7] Lopez-Virella, M. F., P. G. Stone, S. Ellis and J. A. Collwell, Clin. Chem. **23**, 882—884 (1977).
[8] Perédi, J., M. Somogyi and M. Jeránek, Olaj Szappan Kozmetika **26**, 11 (1977).
[9] Perédi, J., M. Somogyi and M. Jeránek, Acta aliment. **7**, 279 (1978).
[10] Eleftheriades, P., J. Perédi, M. Jeránek and M. Somogyi, Olaj Szappan Kozmetika **29**, 11 (1980).
[11] Sachs, L., Applied statistics. A handbook of techniques. Springer-Verlag, Berlin, Göttingen, Heidelberg 1984.
[12] Zöllner, N., and K. Krisch, Z. ges. exp. Med. **135**, 545—562 (1962).

Dr. Á. J. N. Zsinka (present address: Central Food Research Institute, H-1525 Budapest, Herman Ottó ut. 15), Dr. K. Lindner-Szotyori and Prof. Dr. Gy. Biró, National Institute of Food Hygiene and Nutrition, H-1097 Budapest, Gyáli ut. 3/a, and Dr. J. Perédi, Vegetable Oil and Detergent Research Institute, H-1106 Budapest, Maglódi ut. 6, Hungary

Received April 10, 1987

Rezensionen

Chemistry and Physics of Baking. Materials, Processes and Products. Proceedings of an International Symposium, The School of Agriculture, Sutton Bonington, 10th—12th April 1985. Herausgegeben von J. M. V. Blanshard, P. J. Frazier und T. Galliard. 276 Seiten, zahlr. Abb. und Tab. The Royal Society of Chemistry, London 1986. Preis: 39,50 £; 71,— $.

Die Entwicklungsgeschichte des Backprozesses reicht mindestens 6000 Jahre zurück, und die Backwarenindustrie nimmt vom Umfang und Wert der Produktion her einen sehr hohen volkswirtschaftlichen Rang ein. Technologisch gesehen, ist sie jedoch ein schlafender Riese. Die handwerklichen Traditionen sind nicht abgestreift, die Material- und Prozeßkenntnisse lückenhaft, dem aktuellen Vergleich mit denen von Hochtechnologien nicht standhaltend. In erster Linie betrifft dies die bio- und physikochemischen Grundlagen, speziell die für die Prozeßgestaltung und Produkteigenschaften bestimmenden molekularen Gegebenheiten und Vorgänge. Das, zunehmender ökonomischer Druck und die sich aus wandelnden Verzehrsgewohnheiten, Versorgungssituationen und ernährungsphysiologischen Bedürfnissen ergebenden Herausforderungen waren für die Sektion Lebensmittelchemie der Royal Society of Chemistry und die Abteilung für angewandte Biochemie und Lebensmittelchemie der Landwirtschaftlichen Fakultät an der Universität Nottingham Veranlassung, im April 1985 ein Symposium zu veranstalten, auf dem mit einer international gut besetzten Rednerliste, Vergleich und Integration suchend, 20, hier wiedergegebene Vorträge gehalten und diskutiert worden sind. Sieben davon befassen sich mit den wesentlichsten Komponenten von Backwaren (Stärke, Nichtstärke-Polysaccharide, Proteine, Lipide, Enzyme, Wasser, Hefe, Emulgatoren und andere Backhilfsmittel), sechs mit fundamentalen Wechselwirkungen von Teiginhaltsstoffen im Knet- und Backprozeß sowie bei der Lagerung, ihren Konsequenzen und den Möglichkeiten ihrer Kontrolle und Steuerung, und vier handeln laufende oder sich abzeichnende Prozeß- und Produktentwicklungen bzw. -optimierungen einschließlich der Züchtung neuer, der Qualitätsverbesserung von Backwaren dienender Weizensorten ab. Jedem Vortrag ist ein Literaturverzeichnis, und am Ende ist ein Sachwortregister beigefügt. Diskussionsbeiträge sind leider weder festgehalten, noch zusammenfassend ausgewertet. So bleibt es dem Leser überlassen, aus hervorragenden Bestandsaufnahmen und einer Reihe von Denkanstößen die mit dem Symposium angestrebten Schlußfolgerungen selbst zu ziehen und sei es nur die, daß umwälzende Technologien wohl auch künftig oder zumindest vorerst nicht zu erwarten sind.

B. Gassmann

Alter und Ernährung, enteral and parenteral. Neunzehntes Bad Sodener Geriatrisches Gespräch 8. Mai 1987. Herausgegeben von V. Böhlau. 116 Seiten, 11 Abb., 22 Tab. Schattauer, Stuttgart, New York 1988. Preis: 52.— DM.

In 7 Übersichtsvorträgen werden Fragen der Altersernährung angesprochen. Sie beziehen sich auf Grundlagen der Ernährung im Alter generell und auf die Diättherapie, auf die Grundlagen der parenteralen und auf die der Sondenernährung. Einbezogen werden allgemeine Fragen des höheren Alters, besonders die Forderung nach Gesundheit der Senioren, nach der altersgerechten Wohnung, nach der altersgerechten Ernährung. Widersprüchlich wird die Frage des Eiweißbedarfs diskutiert, einerseits die Forderung auf 1,2—1,4 g, bei kompletter parenteraler Ernährung sogar 1,6 g täglich, andererseits werden 0,8—1,0 g als ausreichend angesehen. Doch sind dabei individuelle Situationen zu berücksichtigen. Wichtig ist sicherlich der Hinweis, daß bei sehr alten Menschen ansonsten aktuelle Gesichtspunkte der Ernährungsprophylaxe nicht mehr relevant sind. Interessant sind Erwägungen zum Thema „Altern — eine Last?". Dabei wird z. B. auf die frühere Bedeutung der Familie für die Fürsorge um den alten Menschen hingewiesen, während heute die soziale Sicherheit im Alter als Aufgabe der Gesellschaft gesehen wird. Es würde dabei ein übermäßiges Anspruchsdenken in der Bevölkerung gezüchtet. Eine Korrektur erscheint angezeigt bezüglich der hier gegebenen Darstellung, daß die WHO die Gesundheit als Zustand eines objektiven und subjektiven Wohlbefindens in körperlicher, seelischer und geistiger Hinsicht beschreiben würde. Richtig heißt es vielmehr: „Gesundheit ist der Zustand des vollständigen körperlichen, geistigen und sozialen Wohlbefindens und nicht nur das Freisein von Krankheit oder Gebrechen". Insgesamt ein anregendes Büchlein.

H. Haenel

Die Nahrung 32 (1988) 9, 823—830

Research Institute for Food Industry* and National Center for Scientific Researches**, Havana, Cuba

Analysis of natural citrus aqueous essences

J. Pino*, A. Rosado** and R. Baluja**

Commercially produced natural citrus aqueous essences obtained from orange, grapefruit, lemon and lime were qualitatively analyzed by GC-MS system. The major and most of the minor components had been previously isolated from these fruits. Also some minor components, not previously found were identified in this study.

Introduction

Natural citrus essences are distilled aqueous solutions of the more volatile components from the corresponding citrus juices. Commercially they are added to concentrated citrus juice products to impart fresh fruit flavor that was lost during the concentration process and not restored by addition of peel oil. Essences may be collected from fresh juice by partial distillation prior to juice evaporation or by condensation of volatiles from early stages of evaporation with the aid of an aroma recovery unit [1].

Although natural aqueous essences are recovered during the concentration of all major citrus juices, orange essence is the most important and most widely used citrus essence. The identification of the volatile constituents of orange aqueous essence has been a subject of considerable research since the development of gas-liquid chromatography (GLC) and its combination with mass spectrometry (GC-MS) as analytical techniques for the rapid evaluation of essential oils and essences [2—7], but there have been few comparable studies on other citrus essences [8—10].

In the present study, natural aqueous essences from orange, grapefruit, lemon and lime were qualitatively analyzed using a GC-MS system.

Material and methods

Natural citrus aqueous essences were obtained from a taste essence recovery unit during the production of concentrated juice from Valencia oranges, Duncan grapefruits, Persian limes and Eureka lemons in a local factory in Matanzas, Cuba.

Two liters of aqueous essences were saturated with sodium chloride and extracted three times with methylene chloride [2]. The combined extracts were dried with sodium sulfate and concentrated to small volume at 45 °C with a 15 cm Vigreux column.

GLC analyses were made on a Packard-Becker 419 gas chromatograph using FID detector and equipped with a 0,25 mm i.d. by 30 m UCON LB 550X glass capillary column. The oven temperature was kept at 70 °C for 6 min and then programmed to 220 °C at 5 °C/min with an argon flow of 0,8 ml/min.

GC-MS analyses were made on a Jeol JMS-DX 300 equipped with a 0,25 mm i.d. by 25 m FFAP fused silica capillary column or OV-17 fused silica capillary column. The split ratio was 1:20. The injector, inlet and ion source temperatures were 220 °C and the ion energy was 70 eV.

The qualitative analysis was made by comparing mass spectras as well as retention times with those of known compounds or by comparing mass spectras with reported data [11—15].

Results and discussion

Fig. 1—4 show the reconstructed chromatograms obtained by recording the total ion current. These chromatograms give an indication of the number and amount of the volatile components in the natural citrus aqueous essences, where the most complex composition belong to orange and the less complex composition seemes to be grapefruit aqueous essence.

The major organic components of the citrus aqueous essences are ethanol, methanol and acetaldehyde, which are not quantitatively recovered with the extraction technique used in this study. Other major and minor components were also identified and for other no identified there are described the six main fragments of the mass spectrum.

Orange (Citrus sinensis L. Osbeck)

The chromatogram is indicated in Fig. 1 and the identified components listed in Table 1. A compilation of volatile components found in orange oils, aqueous essence and juice gives 238 components [16]. Although most of the components listed in the TNO compilation were not found in any one study, most were identified more than once as an orange volatiles. Nine of the components identified in this study that had not been previously reported as orange volatiles are acetoin, isoisopulegol, neoisoisopulegol, p-cymen-8-ol, trans and cis carvyl acetate, isopiperitenone, methyl eugenol and estragol. Since neoisopulegol and perilla alcohol had been reported once in orange the present study confirms their presences.

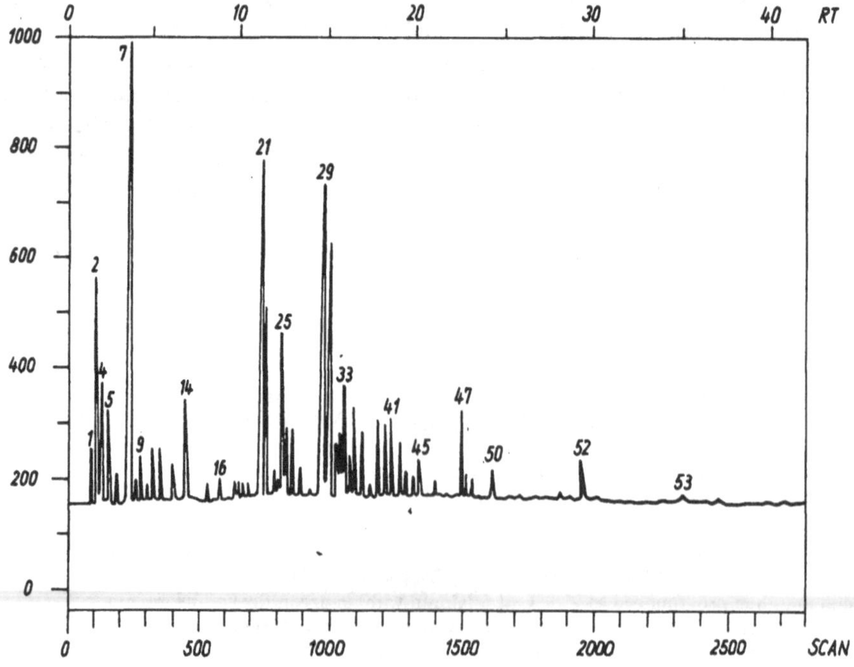

Fig. 1
GC-MS analysis of natural orange aqueous essence. Conditions: FFAP fused silica capillary column from 70—180 °C at 4 °C/min. Flow rate 0.2 ml/min. Injection 0.4 μl with split ratio 1:50

Table 1
Components identified in orange aqueous essence

Peak	Component	Peak	Component
1	ethyl acetate, acetal	29	ethyl 3-hydroxyhexanoate
2	solvent	30	α-terpineol
3	trichloroethylene[b]	31	valencene
4	ethyl butyrate	32	carvone
5	isobutanol	33	geranial
6	$C_6H_{10}O$ 41(100) 42(25) 43(21) 55(22) 56(35) 69(38)	34	trans-carvyl acetate[a]
		35	cis-carvyl acetate[a]
7	limonene, 3-methyl-1-butanol	36	perillaldehyde
8	trans-2-hexenal	37	neryl acetate
9	1-pentanol	38	geranyl acetate
10	acetoin[a]	39	nerol
11	1-octanal	40	isopiperitenone[a]
12	1-penten-3-ol, 2-methyl-3-buten-2-ol	41	trans-carveol
		42	geraniol
13	1-hexanol	43	cis-carveol
14	cis-3-hexen-1-ol	44	$C_{10}H_{16}O$ 41(74) 55(59) 91(100) 109(79) 119(90) 134(89)
15	trans-epoxydihydrolinalool		
16	cis-epoxidihydrolinalool	46	1-p-menthen-9-ol
17	isopulegol	47	$C_{10}H_{18}O_2$ 67(77) 68(95) 79(100) 91(80) 105(77) 119(87)
18	isoisopulegol[a]		
19	neoisopulegol	48	perilla alcohol
20	neoisoisopulegol[a]	49	methyl eugenol[a]
21	linalool	50	octanoic acid
22	1-octanol	51	estragol[a]
23	$C_{10}H_{18}O$ 41(82) 68(73) 69(80) 81(100) 93(78) 121(96)	52	$C_{10}H_{16}O$ 43(74) 62(82) 71(100) 81(62) 82(56) 109(50)
25	terpinen-4-ol	53	nootkatone
26	$C_9H_{18}O_2$ 41(13) 43(73) 71(100) 97(14) 115(21) 158(17)		
27	p-cymen-8-ol		

[a] Not previously identified
[b] possible impurity from solvent

As indicated in Fig. 1, the major isolated components are limonene, 3-methyl-l-butanol, linalool, ethyl 3-hydroxyhexanoate and α-terpineol.

Grapefruit (Citrus paradisi McFadyen)

The chromatogram is shown in Fig. 2 and the list of identified components in Table 2. Among the 121 volatiles recorded by VAN STRATEN et al. [16], only 21 have been found again. Surprisingly, we did not find nootkatone, a typical compound of grapefruit flavour. Tetramethylmethane had not previously been found in citrus. It is not probably an impurity from the solvent and because of its structure, the flavour contribution of this new citrus compound is not significant.

The major isolated components are ethyl acetate, 3-methyl-l-butanol, l-octanol and α-terpineol.

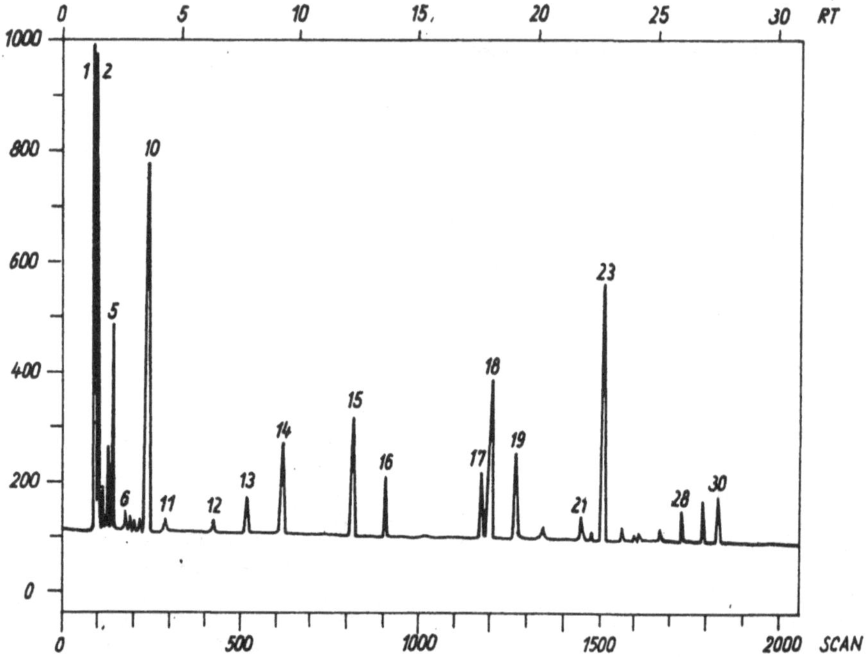

Fig. 2
GC-MS analysis of natural grapefruit aqueous essence. Conditions: FFAP fused silica capillary column at 80 °C for 10 min, 80—200 °C at 4 °C/min. Flow rate 0.4 ml/min. Injection 0.4 µl with split ratio 1:50

Table 2
Components identified in grapefruit aqueous essence

Peak	Component	Peak	Component
1	ethyl acetate	16	cis-epoxydihydrolinalool
2	solvent	17	linalool
3	methyl butyrate	18	1-octanol
4	ethyl butyrate	19	terpinen-4-ol
5	2-methyl propanol	21	neral
7	tetramethylmethane[a]	23	α-terpineol
9	limonene	27	citronelol
10	3-methyl-1-butanol	28	nerol
13	1-hexanol	29	trans carveol
14	cis-3-hexen-1-ol	30	geraniol
15	trans-epoxydihydrolinalool		

[a] Not previously identified

Lemon (Citrus limonun)

Of the four citrus aqueous essences the aroma of lemon essence most resemble the fruit from which it was produced. Table 3 shows the 28 components identified in the chromatogram (Fig. 3). Surprisingly, we did not identify lower carbon chain alcohols than did MOSHONAS et al. [8]. On the other hand many sesquiterpene hydrocarbons have been found, some

Table 3
Components identified in lemon aqueous essence

Peak	Component	Peak	Component
1	solvent	22	neral, trans-carveol
2	tetrachloroethylene[b]	23	geranial
3	α-pinene	24	geraniol
4	β-pinene	25	β-elemene
5	sabinene	26	α-bergamotene
6	β-myrcene	27	β-caryophillene
7	limonene	28	trans-β-farnesene[a]
8	p-cymene	29	α-humulene
9	γ-terpinene	31	$C_{15}H_{24}$ 41(59) 55(24) 69(100) 93(68) 133(26) 161(26)
10	terpinolene	32	α-cubebene
11	trans-epoxydihydrolinalool[a]	33	$C_{15}H_{24}$ 41(27) 91(23) 93(100) 107(24) 109(29) 204(45)
12	cis-epoxydihydrolinalool[a]	34	β-bisabolene
13	1-octanol	35	$C_{15}H_{24}$ 41(64) 55(57) 69(62) 79(44) 93(100) 123(49)
14	$C_{10}H_{18}O$ 41(40) 55(26) 71(36) 93(100) 121(30) 136(25)	36	$C_{15}H_{24}$ 41(52) 68(56) 81(65) 93(70) 105(66) 161(100)
15	sabinene hydrate[a]	37	$C_{15}H_{24}$ 80(28) 93(100) 109(27) 119(27) 121(22) 204(26)
17	linalool	38	γ-elemene[a]
18	borneol[a]		
19	α-terpineol		
20	$C_{10}H_{16}O$ 43(41) 59(100) 79(65) 91(44) 94(74) 119(33)		
21	nerol		

[a] Not previously identified
[b] Possible impurity from solvent

being not identified. Six new components are also described, trans- and cis-epoxydihydrolinalool, sabinene hydrate, borneol, trans β-farnesene and γ-elemene.

The major isolated components are limonene, α-terpineol, β-caryophillene and β-bisabolene.

The contribution of neral and geranial to lemon flavour is unquestionable.

Lime (Citrus aurantifolia Swingle)

The essence of lime is also strongly characteristic of the fruit from which it was produced. The chromatogram is shown in Fig. 4 and the identified components listed in Table 4.

Among the 93 volatiles listed by VAN STRATEN et al. [16], only 26 have been found again. Eight new components are also described, l-pentanol, trans- and cis-carvyl acetate, piperitone, isopiperitenone, trans-β-farnesene, β-cubebene and α-bisabolene.

The major isolated components are limonene, terpinen-4-ol, α-terpineol, neral and geranial.

Neral and geranial undoubtedly contribute to the typical lime flavour, but some other components such as p-cymene and 1,8-cineol largely contribute to the overall impression.

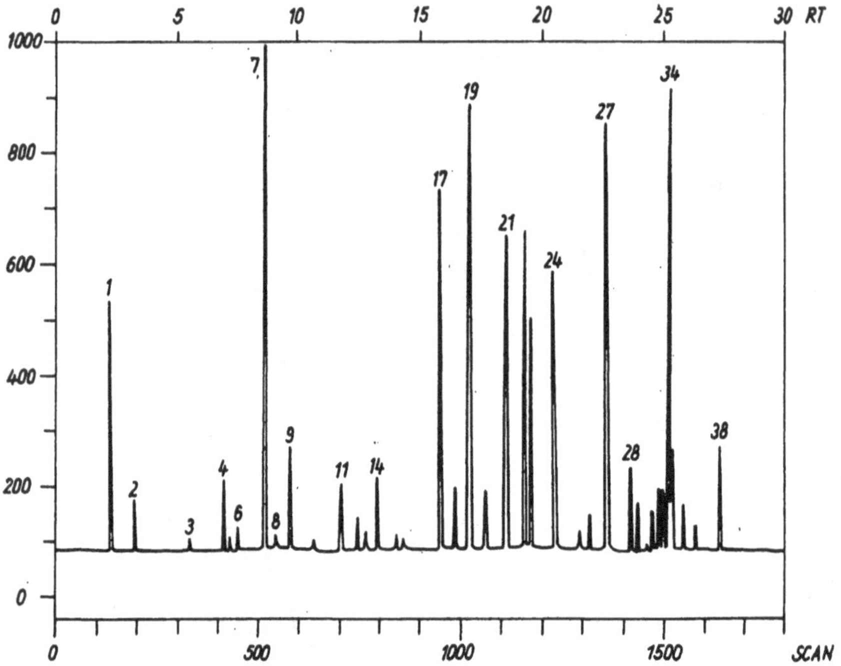

Fig. 3.
GC-MS analysis of natural lemon aqueous essence. Conditions: OV-17 fused silica capillary column from 70—200 °C at 4 °C/min. Flow rate 0.7 ml/min. Injection 0.25 µl with split ratio 1:20

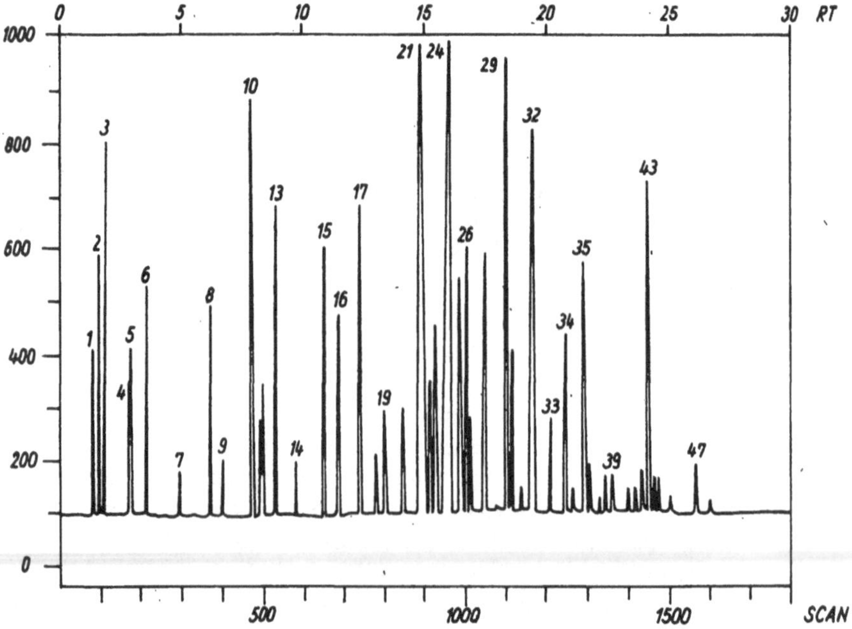

Fig. 4
GC-MS analysis of natural lime aqueous essence. Conditions: OV-17 fused silica capillary column from 70—200 °C at 4 °C/min. Flow rate 0.6 ml/min. Injection 0.3 µl with split ratio 1:20

Table 4
Components identified in lime aqueous essence

Peak	Component	Peak	Component
1	solvent	23	borneol
2	ethyl acetate	24	α-terpineol
3	2-methyl-3-buten-2-ol	25	trans-carvyl acetate[a]
4	1-pentanol	26	$C_{10}H_{14}O$ 43(82) 59(100) 79(56) 94(68) 132(38) 135(38)
5	tetrachloroethylene[b]		
6	3-methyl-2-buten-1-ol	27	cis-carvyl acetate[a]
7	α-pinene	28	neryl acetate
8	β-pinene	29	neral
9	β-myrcene	30	nerol
10	limonene	31	piperitone[a]
11	p-cymene	32	geranial
12	1,8-cineole	33	isopiperitenone[a]
13	γ-terpinene	34	geranyl acetate
14	α-terpinolene	35	α-bergamotene
15	trans-epoxydihydrolinalool	36	$C_{10}H_{16}O$ 43(42) 59(81) 79(97) 91(41) 94(100) 119(41)
16	cis-epoxydihydrolinalool		
17	linalool	38	trans-β-farnesene[a]
18	$C_{10}H_{18}O$ 43(28) 77(30) 91(31) 93(100) 121(21) 136(26)	39	$C_{10}H_{16}O$ 43(34) 59(100) 79(79) 91(46) 94(87) 119(42)
19a	fenchyl alcohol	41	β-cubebene[a]
19b	$C_{10}H_{16}O$ 41(45) 79(47) 81(38) 91(100) 119(94) 134(79)	42	α-bisabolene[a]
		43	β-bisabolene
20	$C_{10}H_{18}O$ 41(43) 43(55) 92(81) 93(100) 119(63) 134(60)	44	$C_{15}H_{22}O$ 41(63) 55(55) 69(59) 79(42) 93(100) 123(44)
21	terpinen-4-ol	45	$C_{10}H_{16}O_2$
22	$C_{10}H_{16}O$ 41(60) 69(100) 84(85) 91(53) 119(64) 134(42)	47	γ-elemene

[a] Not previously identified
[b] Possible impurity from solvent

Zusammenfassung

J. PINO, A. ROSADO und R. BALUJA: Analyse von natürlichen, wäßrigen Citrus-Essenzen

Kommerziell hergestellte natürliche, wäßrige Citrus-Essenzen aus Orangen, Grapefruit, Zitronen und Limonen werden qualitativ mittels eines GC-MS-Systems analysiert. Die Hauptkomponenten und die meisten der Nebenbestandteile wurden bereits aus diesen Früchten isoliert. Einige Nebenkomponenten, die vorher noch nicht gefunden wurden, konnten in dieser Studie identifiziert werden.

Резюме

И. ПИНО, А. РОЗАДО и Р. БАЛУЯ: Анализ натуральных водних цитрусовых эссенций

Промышленно полученные натуральные водные цитрусовые эссенции из апельсин, грейпфрутов, лимонов и сладких лимонов подвергались качественному определению с помощью системы газовой хроматографии и массовой спектроскопии. Основные компоненты и большинство побочных частей из этих фруктов уже изолировались. Удалось идентифицировать в этой работе некторые побочные компоненты, которые раньше не были обнаружены.

References

[1] MANNHEIM, C., and N. PASSY, Proc. Int. Soc. Citriculture **3**, 756 (1977).
[2] WOLFORD, R., G. ALBERDING and J. ATTAWAY, J. agric. Food Chem. **10**, 297 (1962).
[3] WOLFORD, R., J. ATTAWAY and L. BARABAS, Proc. Fla. State Hort. Soc. **78**, 268 (1965).
[4] SCHULTZ, T., D. BLACK, J. BOMBEN, T. MON and R. TERANISHI, J. Food Sci. **32**, 698 (1967).
[5] MOSHONAS, M., and P. SHAW, J. Food Sci. **38**, 360 (1973).
[6] SHAW, P., and M. MOSHONAS, Proc. Fla. State Hort. Soc. **87**, 305 (1974).
[7] JOHNSON, J., and J. VORA, Food Technol. **37**, 92 (1983).
[8] MOSHONAS, M., and P. SHAW, J. agric. Food Chem. **19**, 119 (1971).
[9] MOSHONAS, M., and P. SHAW, J. agric. Food Chem. **20**, 70 (1972).
[10] MOSHONAS, M., and P. SHAW, J. agric. Food Chem. **20**, 1029 (1972).
[11] VON SYDOW, E., Acta chem. scand. **17**, 2504 (1963).
[12] VON SYDOW, E., Acta chem. scand. **18**, 1099 (1964).
[13] VON SYDOW, E., Acta chem. scand. **19**, 2083 (1965).
[14] MOSHONOS, M., and E. LUND, Flavour Ind. **1**, 375 (1970).
[15] STENHAGEN, E., S. ABRAHAMSON and F. MCLAFFERTY, Registry of mass spectral data. John and Sons, Inc., New York 1974.
[16] VAN STRATEN, S., and H. MAARSE, Volatile compounds in food, CIVO-TNO, Zeist-NL, 1983.

Dr. JORGE A. PINO, Research Institute for Food Industry (IIIA) Ave. Rancho Boyeros km $3^1/_2$, Cerro, Havana, Çuba

Received April 13, 1987

Die Nahrung 32 (1988) 9, 831—838

Central Institute of Nutrition in Potsdam-Rehbrücke (Director: Prof. Dr. H. SCHMANDKE), Academy of Sciences of the GDR

Review article

Is the variational scope of individual sensitivity given enough consideration in evaluation of risks caused by toxicological substances in food?

D. W. R. BLEYL

The contemporary concept of evaluation of risks with humans caused by xenobiotics in food is critically reviewed. In this context it is pointed out that epidemiologic studies, in most cases, give little reliable evidence only. Mankind's risk factors are of a multi-dimensional composition, depending on genetic aspects and the differring health and nutrition statuses of the individuals. This leads to an enormously wide scope of variations in the individual sensitivity to xenobiotics. Contemporary knowledge leaves the question open, whether predisposed population groups are always sufficiently protected by the level of the permissible amount of xenobiotics.

The basic concept of nutritional toxicology concerning the admission of xenobiotics has not changed during the last 30 years [1, 2]. It is based on the hypothesis that all substances have toxic effects on the mammalian organism, if exceeding a threshold dosage (PARACELSUS, 1538). This hypothesis leads to two tasks concerning toxicologic risk assessment with humans:

— the detection of possible effects of substances (so-called characterization, which, for ethical reasons, is performed on laboratory animals only),
— the assessment of the threshold dosage of a substance which is not exceeding a very low, acceptable, or reasonable risk for the human individual during a life-long exposition, and which takes into consideration all hitherto known facts (actual risk assessment). Qualitatively seen, this mostly is understood as involving an incident frequency of 10^{-6} and below [3, 30].

Toxicity tests in experiments on animals for the permission of xenobiotics are all based on a one-dimensional risk assessment. Without undergoing preliminary treatment, healthy animals of the same age, sex and breed of, if possible, two or more species, one of which should not be a rodent, are exposed in groups to different doses of a single substance or a mixture of substances under, if possible, precisely defined and optimal conditions. Suitable criteria help to detect the maximum amount of a substance that is tolerated by laboratory animals (no-observed-effect level). Concerning the necessary scope of investigations on animals, our attention should rather focus on the no-observed, than on the observed parameters, since certain xenobiotics sometimes produced unexpected effects in the past.

"As a rule, you only find what you are looking for. And you are only looking for what is known. Taking this for granted, we would have to presuppose that all possible, harmful effects which might occur under any conditions are known already" [4]. The rightly debated problem of species-bound specific criteria (caecomegalia, osmotically conditioned diarrhoea) principally can only be overcome, if different species of animals are used. This method is advisable anyhow in the case of caecectomized mice [5] and diabetic rats [53], where the influence of the caecal flora after Hg-exposition cannot be interpreted without special investigations. The evaluation of risks would be optimized essentially, if the reversibility of the effects of xenobiotics in animal experiments were tested in addition. Most widely reproducible results can be guaranteed if the various tests (Fig. 1) are performed in accordance with GLP standards [6, 7]. This, on the other hand, does not mean at all that the derived no-observed-effect level represents a constant figure. On the contrary, it is dependent on a number of parameters: the species, the breed, the sex and age of the tested animals, the duration of the experiment, the animals' food, and many other environmental factors [8]. As is easily proved by theoretical examples, the choice of the random test extention plays a further role [3, 9]. In that context, the dependency on errors of the 1st and the 2nd category is of essential importance. Hence, it would be correct for the experimentator to fix, on the basis of medical considerations, the significant difference alpha for the individual criteria which have to be defined. This would give a clue to the extension of the random tests needed when considering a given probability of error. Due to labour technology and cost factors, toxicologic experiments on animals can only be performed within a rather limited scope. As a result, the no-observed-effect level defined by the comparison of average values, and depending on the choice of dosage gradation, is more or less close to the theoretical value. The application of mathematical models for the description of the detected dosage-effect

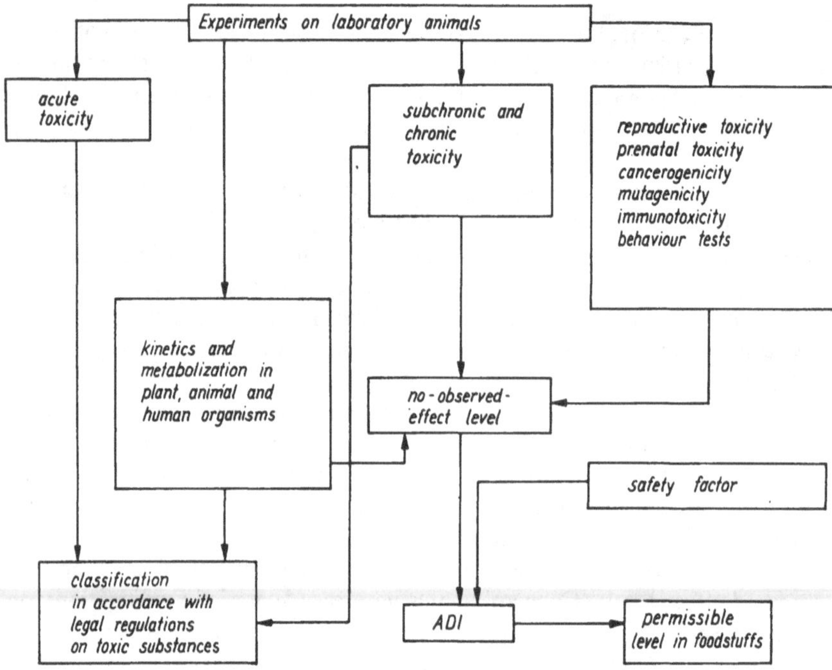

Fig. 1
One-dimensional risk assessment for the deduction of tolerance value

relations can reduce the importance of this inedequacy, since it allows for the mathematical assessment of the no-observed-effect level between the dosage groupings [9, 10].

The extrapolation of results gained in animal experiments on humans presents the real problem with regard to toxicological risk evaluation. It is justified by fundamental considerations on model tests [11, 12]. But, as a rule, even the necessary use of a metabolically best suited test animal for the testing of a substance X in praxi depends on the local conditions of the testing institute and is reduced to the use of one and the same breed of test animals over a couple of years. Extrapolation of animal test results on humans therefore involves a decisive qualitative leap. Apart from physiological and specific differences of the species, the multi-dimensional influence of variables on the penetration and expressivity of xenobiotic effects has to be taken into consideration. These variables are, amongst others, differentiated food and disease patterns, differences in life expectancy and reproduction behaviour, the occurrence of stress situations, metabolic and physiologic differences, and the possibility of a continuous exposition to a multitudiny of xenobiotics (ca. 50—70,000) from various sources over the whole life of the individual or over several generations [13].

The concept of risk evaluation for 30 years now has provided for the introduction of a safety factor of mostly 1:100 [1, 2]. Differences in sensitivity between the test animals and humans, and the individual sensitivity variations within the human population [14] are each given a quota of 10. Even if the WHO in certain cases recommends other safety factors (1:25 with chlorfenvinphos as a cholinesterase blocking agent [15]; but 1:1000 with captan, due to prenatal toxicological effects [16]), and thus varies the procedure occasionally, it cannot be denied that the whole approach is rather pragmatic. Theoretical calculations have shown that a constant safety factor can have different degrees of effectivity. These calculations are based on the inclination function of the dosage-effect relation found in experiments. Fig. 2 shows this function in 3 theoretical substances. It can be seen that the safety factor loses effectivity with a decrease of the slope function. This fact deserves positive attention. A complete answer to all the questions cannot be given yet, even if comparative kinetic investigations are involved more [17—19].

Even in the future, toxicological evaluation of risks with humans will only be possible on

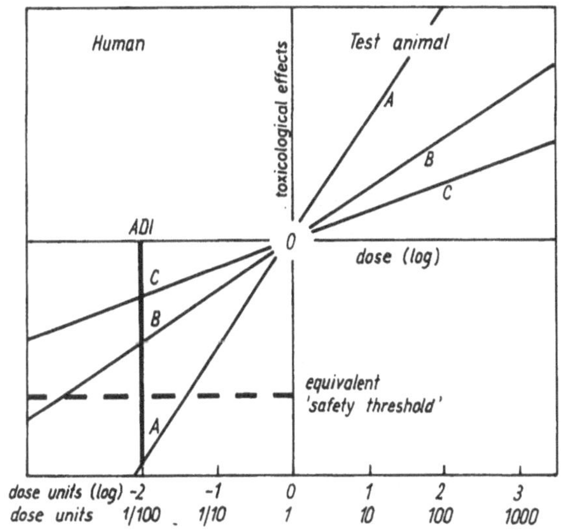

Fig. 2
Relation between applied safety factor taken from 100 concerning the extrapolation of results of animal experiments on humans and indicating the safety threshold gained in dependency on the inclination function of the dosage — effect — relation

the basis of animal toxicity tests. Therefore, the effectivity of this method can only be tested if unprejudiced analyses of the epidemiologic situation are performed. It has to be taken for granted that human life is never free of risk [20]. The potential, partial risk that possibly results out of the xenobiotic exposition from food can be defined only, if a suitable and precise testing method is available which allows for the differentiation from other sources of risk. Today, do we really have such a prerequisite? Apart from some exceptions (Minamata disease [21], illicit use of dressed grain [22], consumption of rape seed oil contaminated with aniline [23]), and a conspicuous spreading of certain diseases due to the exposition to notoriously suspect substances (aflatoxin ingestion and incidence rate of liver cancer in Kenia [24], correlation between used nitrate fertilizers and the occurrence of stomach carcinome in Chile [25, 26], 'Balkanese nephropathy' [27], cancer of oesophagus due to the eating broken fern in Japan [28]) there are no further findings from epidemiological studies in the industrialized countries given reference to toxicological risks for humans [29].

The simple question to be put now is, whether these 'negative results' can be taken as pieces of absolute evidence, thus denying the necessity of any further activities. This opinion is almost exclusively expressed in contemporary literature. In its support, historic evidence and comparisons with other risks are utilized. According to ELTON [30], mankind have found their present food by trial and error. There is no guarantee that our traditional foodstuff does not present any toxicological risk factors. Comparisons of non-quantified nutritional risk studies with statistical mortality risk studies concerning various factors of the ways of life in industrialized countries [31—33] are, to a certain extent, quite impressive, especially if the latter are used to deduct an individual annual risk of 10^{-5}, which is taken as acceptable in the face of an average life expectancy of 70—75 years [30]. GRICE [20] refers to rough quantitative readings and general observations stating that the population, on the one hand, is ready to go in for a risk, e.g. by smoking, drinking, or sports activities, if they, on the other hand, can achieve 'gains' out of doing so. This comparison is not permissible, because the fixing of risks caused by toxicological substances in food is part of the state's responsibility. According to DARBY [34], the upper limit of the total risk from the intake of food should not exceed the risk level of natural diseases.

Contrary to experimental analyses which only accept 'negative results' within a network of several test systems [35], so far, there has been almost no attempt to probe into the evidence of epidemiological studies. It should be clear that, nowadays, acutely lethal effects by xenobiotics in foodstuff can only be expected if the xenobiotics are applied wrongly. The question is: Are these the only effects to be considered? The poignancy of the statistical mortality risks mentioned above is just based on the fact that, e.g. any traffic accident can be analyzed precisely with regard to time, place, persons involved, persons killed, etc. But the exposure of a certain human or a human average (referring to the temporal process) to a substance X and its sources can only be assessed in rough estimates. Let us assume that a substance X produces effects which, as is demonstrated by the occurrence of cancer of the oesophagus after the consumption of fern [28], or the transplacental carcinogenesis of diethystilbestrole [36, 37], probably only become evident in a population after 10 or more years. In such a case, we have to ask ourselves which chances those latent periods give to us to plausibly demonstrate the relation of cause and effect, as well as the independence from other variables. But only after such long periods epidemiological studies have any power of evidence [29]. According to KEWITZ [38], the understanding of physicians has to be deepened generally to make them see that this gives them a new task in addition to their daily diagnostic work. Referring to the deduction of the ADI-factor, it has to be added that, for methodological reasons, epidemiology basically has confined itself to the detection of environmental factors as the reasons or accessory conditions for diseases. So far, apart from fluorine, threshold levels as the reasons for certain effects in a population have hardly ever been the subject matter of systematic research [39].

There cannot be any doubt that the detection of xenobiotic effects in humans makes it immensely important to know about the changes brought forth and their characteristics. Research into the epidemiologically extremely rare prenatal effects (A-, micro-, and phocomelia) caused by thalidomide on ca. 40 children could establish the probability of the relation of cause and effect within half a year [40]. But, as has to be concluded from animal experiments, most cases only produce relatively 'unspecific changes' at the end of the time of exposure. These changes do not stand out very clearly, or even not at all, against the background of the total situation consisting of multiple in- and extrinsic factors. In many cases, late damages, e.g. liver cirrhosis, of manifold origins can be found as well. The same holds for the hyperkinetic syndrome with 1—15% of American children. Probable reasons, such as natal traumas, smoking during pregnancy, environmental lead contamination, or allergies against certain foodstuffs, are being discussed [41—43]. Another typical example of this present situation is contamination with cadmium from various sources. Meanwhile, this has reached such a level that between 10,000 and 100,000 citizens of the Federal Republic of Germany are supposed to be susceptible to kidney disorders [44]. To sum it up, we have to conclude that, at present, we do not have the precise method to measure and assess the wide scope of possible toxicological risks. This holds for the assessment of evidence from epidemiological studies, too.

The ADI-value derived from the no-observed-effect level and the safety factor of any food substance has to be regarded as a crude indication concerning the quantitative amount which might be tolerated safely by humans. Therefore it seems necessary now to purposefully acquire knowledge on the scope of variations in the individual sensitivity found amongst the human population. Fragmentary clues have so far been provided by biochemical and kinetic studies. They demonstrate quantitative dispersions which by far exceed those of the groups of tested animals, or which are above the respective proportional range provided for the extrapolation of animal test results on humans. With humans, the individual binding of benzo(a)pyrene to the DNS of explanted bronchial tissue varies up to 75-fold [45], in the case of colon tissue the ratio is 100-fold even [46]. Comparable results are available concerning the metabolization of N-nitrosamines [47]. Here, parallel testing has shown an interindividual range of dispersion which was 33 times higher with humans than with mice, rats, or bovines [48].

This is due to genetic aspects (e.g. so-called excessive and poor metabolizers [49], polymorphisms of the cytochrome P-450 [50], or the Ah-locus [51]). Besides, enzymopathies have to be mentioned, too. The National Academy of Sciences of the USA has listed a total of 92 of those [52]. Their hereditary carriers display a more or less strong pre-disposition if exposed to xenobiotics. Apart from these genetic factors, the heterogeneous field of the respective health and nutrition status of the population, above all, modifies toxicological effects [53]. In our own experiments, epidemiologically relevant conditions were modelled [53]. In those, to give an example, the penetration of prenatal toxicological effects in the F_1-generation of nullipar females and adult breeding females were shaped differently. Dependence of the metabolism on applied xenobiotics (gamma-HCH and ethylene-thiourea) on the constitutional biotransformatory enzyme pattern could be proved with diabetic as well as with precirrhotic rats. Added to that, diabetic rats showed a decisively higher renale

Hg-accumulation. Prenatal toxicologic investigations could demonstrate practically relevant combination effects of ethanole with other xenobiotics. In any case, the situation of exposing humans to a substance, if compared with standardized laboratory tests on animals, has to be assessed far more heterogeneously. It is permissible to speak of a multi-dimensional risk composition [56].

GEHRING et al. [54] have used theoretical substances to produce very clear graphic schemes on differences which can result from the wide scope of individual sensitivity in the human population. From those graphs they deduce the demand for safety factors of varied levels for the individual xenobiotics. But epidemiologic results do not in all cases confirm the normal distribution that they based their studies on. AL-SHARISTANI et al. [55], when determining the biologic half-time period of methyl mercury in hair samples from 48 patients (without taking account of breast-feeding mothers), found a typical double-peaked curve. This cluster formation has been known before through the lymphocytal AHH-activities within the American population [51].

The diversity and practical relevance of modifying factors on toxicological effects in certain population brackets, so far, has hardly ever been taken into account at all. This problem deserves systematic research by means of epidemiological studies which apply as many non-invasive methods of investigation as possible. Besides, model experiments on animals are needed which purposefully take into account the coergism on a molecular level and the analysis of detoxifying and toxifying mechanisms. It will probably never be quite possible to give a complete individual risk warranty by legal regulations concerning the permissible dosage level of xenobiotics. But here, too, the golden opportunity lies somewhere between ideal and reality. And it has to be found by active work.

Zusammenfassung

D. W. R. BLEYL: Findet die Variationsbreite der individuellen Empfindlichkeit bei der ernährungstoxikologischen Risikoabschätzung genügend Berücksichtigung?

Das Konzept der ernährungstoxikologischen Risikoabschätzung für den Menschen wird einer kritischen Beurteilung unterzogen und in diesem Zusammenhang die zumeist geringe Aussagefähigkeit von epidemiologischen Studien herausgearbeitet. Die vieldimensionale Risikozusammensetzung beim Menschen aufgrund von genetischen Aspekten sowie des unterschiedlichen Gesundheits- und Ernährungszustandes hat als Konsequenz eine enorme Variationsbreite in der individuellen Empfindlichkeit gegenüber Xenobiotica zur Folge. Beim gegenwärtigen Kenntnisstand bleibt offen, ob die festgelegten Toleranzwerte für Xenobiotica für prädisponierte Bevölkerungsgruppen in jedem Fall eine ausreichende Sicherheit darstellen.

Резюме

Д. В. Р. Блейль: Достаточно ли учитывается диапазон вариации индивидуальной чувствительности при оценке гигиено-токсикологического риска?

Концепт гигиено-токсикологической оценки риска питания для человека подвергается критическому анализу и обращается внимание при этом в большинстве случаев небольшую информативную значимость эпидемиологических исследований. Многоразмерый состав факторов риска у человека вследствие генетических аспектов а также различных состояний здоровья и питания приводит в конечном счете ко громадному спектру вариаций в индивидуальной чувствительности ко ксенобиотикам. При настоящем уровне знаний остается открытым, достаточно ли в любом случае предрасположенные группы населения защищены стандартом допущенных ксенобиотиков.

References

[1] General Principles Governing the Use of Food Additives. WHO Techn. Rep. Ser. No. 129 (1957).
[2] Procedures for the Testing of Intentional Food Additives to Establish their Safety for Use. WHO Techn. Ser. No. 144 (1958).
[3] PELIKAN, E. W., in: A Guide to General Toxicology. Ed. by F. HOMBURGER, J. A. HAYES and E. W. PELIKAN, p. 148. Karger, Basel 1983.
[4] NEUBERT, D., AMI-Berichte 1/1980, p. 277. Dietrich Reimer Verlag, Berlin 1980.
[5] SEKO, Y., T. MIURA and M. TAKAHASHI, Acta Pharmacol. Toxicol. **50**, 117 (1982).
[6] FALCONI, G., A. NAVA and A. CUTTICA, in: Animals in Toxicological Research. Ed. by. I. BARTOŠEK, A. GUAITANI and E. PACEI. p. 171. Raven Press, New York 1982.
[7] HAYASHI, Y., Exp. Anim. **31**, 207 (1982).
[8] ELIAS, P. S., in: Chemical toxicology of food. Ed. by C. L. GALLI, R. PAOLETTI and G. VETTORAZZI. p. 47. Elsevier/North-Holland Biomedical Press, Amsterdam 1978.
[9] HOGAN, M. D., and D. G. HOEL, in: Principles and Methods of Toxicology. Ed. by A. W. HAYES. p. 711. Raven press, New York 1982.
[10] SALSBURG, D. S., in: Scientific Considerations in Monitoring and Evaluating Toxicological Research. Ed. by E. J. GRALL. p. 123. Hemisphere Publishing Corporation, Washington 1981.
[11] HEINECKE, H., Ergebn. Exp. Med. **35**, 31 (1980).
[12] HÖRZ, H., Ergebn. Exp. Med. **35**, 13 (1980).
[13] DARBY, W. J., in: Chemical toxicology of food. Ed. by C. L. GALLI, R. PAOLETTI and G. VETTORAZZI. p. 23. Elsevier/North-Holland Biomedical Press, Amsterdam 1978.
[14] BÄR, F., Arch. Toxicol. **32**, 51 (1974).
[15] WHO Food Additives Series No. 1 (1972).
[16] WHO Techn. Rep. Ser. No. 539 (1974).
[17] RUELIUS, H. W., Xenobiotica **17**, 255 (1987).
[18] CALABRESE, E. J., Principles of Animal Extrapolation. John Wiley & Sons, New York 1982.
[19] GILLETTE, J. R., in: Drug Metabolism and Drug Toxicity. Ed. by J. R. MITCHELL and M. G. HORNING. p. 237. Raven Press, New York 1984.
[20] GRICE, H. C., in: Chemical toxicology of Food. Ed. by C. L. GALLI, R. PAOLETTI and G. VETTORAZZI. p. 33. Elsevier/North-Holland Biomedical Press, Amsterdam 1978.
[21] HARADA, Y., Study Group of Minamata Disease, Kumamoto University, Kumamoto 1968.
[22] PARKE, D. V., J. Forensic Sci. Soc. **16**, 189 (1977).
[23] GOULDING, R., in: Food Toxicology — Real or Imaginary Problems? Ed. by G. G. GIBSON and R. WALKER. p. 301. Taylor & Francis, London 1985.
[24] KEEN, P., and P. MARTIN, Tropical Geograph. Med. **23**, 35 (1971).
[25] ZALDIVAR, R., and W. H. WETTERSTRAND, Experientia **31**, 1354 (1975).
[26] ZALDIVAR, R., Experientia **33**, 264 (1977).
[27] CHEMOZEMSKY, I. N., T. S. STOYANOW, T. H. PETKOVA-BOCHAROVA, I. G. NICOLOV, I. V. DRAGANOV, I. I. STOICHEV, Y. TANCHEV, D. NAIDENOV and N. D. KALCHEVA, Int. J. Cancer **19**, 1 (1977).
[28] HIRAYAMA, T., Nutr. Cancer **1**, 67 (1979).
[29] BARKER, D. J. P., in: Food Toxicology — Real or Imaginary Problems? Ed. by G. G. GIBSON and R. WALKER. p. 76. Taylor & Francis, London 1985.
[30] ELTON, G. A. H., in: Food Toxicology — Real or Imaginary Problems? Ed. by G. G. GIBSON and R. WALKER. p. 3. Taylor & Francis, London 1985.
[31] HAENEL, H., Menschliche Ernährung. Sitzungsberichte der AdW der DDR 15N, p. 21 (1980).
[32] DOULL, J., in: Food Safety. Ed. by H. R. ROBERTS. p. 295. John Wiley & Sons, New York 1981.
[33] LEE, B. W., J. Am. Med. Assoc. **246**, 1196 (1981).
[34] DARBY, W. J., in: Chemical toxicology of food. Ed. by C. L. GALLI, R. PAOLETTI and G. VETTORAZZI. p. 23. Elsevier/North-Holland Biomedical Press, Amsterdam 1978.
[35] ANDERSON, D., in: Food Toxicology — Real or Imaginary Problems? Ed. by G. G. GIBSON and R. WALKER. p. 85. Taylor & Francis, London 1985.
[36] ROBBOY, S. J., G. Y. TRUSLOW, J. ANTON and R. M. RICHART, Gynecol. Oncol. **12**, S98 (1981).
[37] CONLEY, G., G. SANT, A. UCCI and H. MITCHESON, J. Am. Med. Assoc. **249**, 1325 (1983).
[38] KEWITZ, H., AMI-Berichte 1/1980, p. 265. Dietrich Reimer Verlag, Berlin 1980.
[39] ADAM, J., in: Biologische Begründung für hygienische Grenzwerte, Martin-Luther-Universität Halle-Wittenberg, Wiss. Beiträge 1982/53 (78), p. 108 (1982).

[40] LENZ, W., Dtsch. Med. Wschr. **86**, 2555 (1961).
[41] RUMMO, J. H., D. K. ROUTH, N. J. RUMMO and J. F. BROWN, Arch. Environ. Health **34**, 120 (1979).
[42] NEEDLEMAN, H. L., CH. GUNNOS, A. LEVITON, R. REED, H. PERESIE, C. MAHER and P. BARRETT, New Engl. J. Med. **300**, 689 (1979).
[43] TRYPHONAS, H., and R. L. TRITES, in: Food Toxicology — Real or Imaginary Problems? Ed. by G. G. GIBSON and R. WALKER. p. 246. Taylor & Francis, London 1985.
[44] EICHLER, W.-D., Gift in unserer Nahrung. Kilda-Verlag, Greven 1982.
[45] HARRIS, C. C., H. AUTRUP, R. CONNOR, L. A. BARRETT, E. M. McDOWELL and B. F. TRUMP, Science **194**, 1067 (1976).
[46] AUTRUP, H., L. A. BARRETT, F. E. JACKSON, M. L. JESUDASON, G. D. STONER, P. PHELPS, B. F. TRUMP and C. C. HARRIS, Gastroenterology **74**, 1248 (1976).
[47] AUTRUP, H., C. C. HARRIS and B. F. TRUMP, Proc. Soc. Exp. Biol. Med. **159**, 111 (1978).
[48] AUTRUP, H., F. C. WEFALD, A. M. JEFFREY, H. TATE, R. D. SCHWARTZ, B. F. TRUMP and C. C. HARRIS, Int. J. Cancer **25**, 293 (1980).
[49] LARREY, D., D. PESSAYRE and J.-P. BENHAMOU, Gastroenterol. Clin. Biol. **9**, 522 (1985).
[50] GUENGERICH, F. P., D. R. UMBENHAUER, P. F. CHURCHILL, P. H. BEAUNE, R. BÖCKER, R. G. KNODELL, M. V. MARTIN and R. S. LLOYD, Xenobiotica **17**, 311 (1987).
[51] KELLERMAN, G., M. LUYTEN-KELLERMAN and C. R. SHAW, New Engl. J. Med. **289**, 934 (1973).
[52] National Academy of Sciences: Special Risk due to Inborn Error of Metabolism. Principles for Evaluating Chemicals in the Environment, Washington, D.C., 1975.
[53] BLEYL, D. W. R., Ernährungstoxikologische Risikobeurteilung heute unter besonderer Berücksichtigung von Ethanolkombinationen, Mobilisation, Alter und speziellen Krankheitsmodellen. Dissertationsschrift B, Humboldt-Universität zu Berlin 1988.
[54] GEHRING, P. J., and K. S. RAO, in: Patt'y industrial hygiene & toxicology. Ed. by H. CRALLEY and B. CRALLEY .p. 567. J. Wiley & Sons, New York 1979.
[55] AL-SHARISTANI, H., and K. M. SHIHAB, Arch. Environ. Health **28**, 342 (1974).
[56] BLEYL, D. W. R., Nahrung **33** (1989), in press.

Dr. sc. D. W. R. BLEYL, Central Institute of Nutrition, Arthur-Scheunert-Allee 114—116, Bergholz-Rehbrücke, DDR-1505

Received April 16, 1987

Die Nahrung 32 (1988) 9, 839—854

Martin-Luther-Universität Halle-Wittenberg, Biotechnikum,
WB Mikrobiologie, Halle, DDR

Die Bedeutung der Wachstumskinetik und Produktbildung für Auswahl und Einsatz von Starterkulturen in der Milchwirtschaft

E. Jöx, A. Unger und H. Weide

Die Aktivität einer Starterkultur (Milchsäure- und Aromaproduktion) ist abhängig von der Konstanz der Zusammensetzung dieser Mischpopulation und von ihrem optimalen Wachstum in verschiedenen Phasen des Fermentationsprozesses. Die Wachstumsparameter spezifische Wachstumsrate (μ), maximale spezifische Wachstumsrate (μ_{max}), Teilungsrate (v), Verdopplungszeit (t_d) und Halbsättigungskonstante (K_s) eines jeden Einzelstammes sind Grundlage für die Stabilität einer Starterkultur und sollten deshalb bei der Herstellung (Neukombination) von Starterkulturen berücksichtigt werden.

Die Wachstumskinetik von Reinkulturen und Mischpopulationen ausgewählter Milchsäurebakterien wird untersucht und die Bedeutung der Wachstumsparameter μ_{max} und K_s von Einzelstämmen für die Starterkulturenherstellung erörtert. Die Analyse des Wachstums und der Produktbildung von Einzel- und Mischpopulationen in rekonstituierter Magermilch unter Berücksichtigung praxisrelevanter Milieufaktoren (pH, Temperatur, Sauerstoff) bietet Möglichkeiten zur Prozeßsteuerung und Optimierung der Produktsynthese (Milchsäure, Diacetyl).

Einleitung

Als Starterkulturen für die Milchwirtschaft haben Milchsäurebakterien der Familien *Streptococcaceae* und *Lactobacillaceae* bisher die größte Bedeutung. Sie werden gezielt als Rein- oder Mischkulturen den zu fermentierenden Materialien zugesetzt. Die Stabilität von Starterkulturen ist eine der wichtigsten biologischen Voraussetzungen für hohe Produktionssicherheit und konstante Qualitätsparameter der Produkte. Derzeit bestehen jedoch sowohl bei der Auswahl bzw. Eignungsprüfung von Stämmen für eine Starterkultur als auch bei deren Einsatz als Mischpopulation im Produktionsprozeß noch zahlreiche Probleme wie z. B.:

— Erhaltung der Säurungsaktivität und Aromabildung über einen möglichst langen Zeitraum,
— Veränderung der Zusammensetzung der Mischpopulation zugunsten der Säurebildner,
— Wachstumshemmung durch
  - nichtoriginäre Hemmstoffe (Antibiotika, Reinigungsmittelrückstände ...),
  - Kontaminationskeime (Hefen, Schimmelpilze ...),
  - Infektion durch Bakteriophagen,
  - Bildung verschiedener Bacteriocine.

Die Möglichkeiten der Genetik, einschließlich der Gentechnik [1—4] zur Schaffung von Hochleistungsstämmen mit günstigen, industriell verwertbaren Eigenschaften wie Phagenresistenz, Antibiotikaresistenz, hohe Produktivität usw. werden bereits umfassend geprüft. Andererseits ist jedoch — nach wie vor — die Kenntnis verschiedener Wachstumsparameter eine grundlegende Voraussetzung für die Stammauswahl. Säurebildung, Proteolyse, Lipolyse und Aromabildung stehen ja — als gütebestimmende Parameter — im Zusammenhang mit der Energiegewinnung und dem Wachstum der Mikroorganismen. Von Bedeutung sind Teilungsrate (v), spezifische Wachstumsrate (μ), maximale spezifische Wachstumsrate (μ_{max}), Verdopplungszeit (t_d), Halbsättigungskonstante (K_s) etc., die dann übersichtlich katalogisiert zur Charakterisierung der Stämme herangezogen werden können [5]. Beziehungen zwischen mikrobiellem Wachstum und Produktbildung wurden bereits an einer Reihe von Starterkulturen untersucht [6—10]. Es sind jedoch kaum Hinweise darüber bekannt, daß Stämme von Starterkulturen grundsätzlich nach ihren Wachstumsparametern charakterisiert oder ausgewählt werden. Die nachfolgend beschriebenen Ergebnisse zur Wachstumskinetik und Produktbildung von Einzel- und Mischkulturen für die Sauerrahmbutterherstellung unter Berücksichtigung praxisrelevanter Milieufaktoren (pH, Temperatur, Sauerstoff) sollen auf entsprechende Möglichkeiten hinweisen.

Material und Methoden

Organismen und Nährmedien

Zwei Stämme der Gattung *Leuconostoc* (L.), *L. citrovorum* 1 und *L. citrovorum* 78/80/L4/81 sowie ein Stamm der Gattung *Streptococcus* (Sc.) mit der Bezeichnung *Sc. cremoris* Scc_{77}/L4/81 sind handelsübliche Säureweckertypen, die vom VEB OSTRA, Dresden, DDR, in lyophilisierter Form geliefert werden. Als Mischkulturen wurden eine L-Kultur R23 vom VEB WTÖZ der Milchindustrie der DDR, Oranienburg, und eine vor jedem Hauptversuch von uns hergestellte Mischkultur eingesetzt, die aus 80% *Sc. cremoris* Scc_{77}/L4/81 und 20% *L. citrovorum* 78/80/L4/81 bestand. Als Medien zur Ermittlung der Wachstumsparameter v, μ, μ_{max} und K_s diente Nährbouillon II (2,5% Nährbouillon I, 0,5% Hefeextrakt, 0,15% Natriumacetat, 0,05% Ascorbinsäure, ad 1000 ml aqua dest. mit unterschiedlichen Lactosekonzentrationen: 3%, 0,5%, 0,4%, der o.g. Starterkulturen in rekonstituierter Magermilch (Magermilchpulver, sprühgetrocknet, VEB Dauermilchwerk Stendal, DDR) durchgeführt.

Vor- und Hauptkultur

Die Anzucht der Vorkultur erfolgte gemäß den Anwendungsrichtlinien des Herstellerbetriebes VEB OSTRA, Dresden, mit resuspendiertem Lyophilisat bei 23 ... 25 °C für maximal 24 h im Wasserbad. Die Vorkultur (Inoculum) der Einzelkulturen wurde bei 30 °C 24 h und die später untersuchten Mischkulturen bei 21 °C bebrütet. Die Einsaatmenge im Hauptversuch betrug 2 ... 5%. Alle Hauptkulturen wurden in 500 ml-Rundkolben mit 200 ml Arbeitsvolumen bei variierter Lactosekonzentration angesetzt. Um den Einfluß des Sauerstoffs auf Wachstum und Produktbildung zu testen, wurde in einigen Versuchsserien je eine Kultur im nicht bewegten Standkolben und eine Parallele als Schüttelkultur unter sonst gleichen Bedingungen hergestellt. Bei der Schüttelkultur kam die elektronische Schüttelmaschine vom Typ THYS3 (Reziprokschüttler), Hersteller VEB MLW Labortechnik Ilmenau, DDR, zur Anwendung.

Bestimmung des Bakterienwachstums

Die Bestimmung des Bakterienwachstums in Nährbouillon II erfolgte nach der indirekten Methode photometrisch mit dem Spektralkolorimeter „Spekol 10" vom VEB Carl Zeiss Jena, DDR, (Wellenlänge 500 nm). Die Keimzahlbestimmung in rekonstituierter Magermilch wurde nach dem KOCH'schen Plattenverfahren durchgeführt. Aus den jeweilig erhaltenen Wachstumskurven wurden unter Bezugnahme der Exponentialphase die Teilungsrate (v) graphisch bzw. nach der Formel:

$$v = \frac{\mathrm{ld}\, N - \mathrm{ld}\, N_0}{t - t_0} \qquad (1)$$

ermittelt und daraus die Wachstumsrate μ nach der Formel

$$\mu = \ln 2\nu \tag{2}$$

näherungsweise berechnet.

Bestimmung des Sauerstoffverbrauchs

Durch die amperometrische Sauerstoffpartialdruckmessung (pO_2) des Gelöstsauerstoffs im Nährmedium mittels membranüberzogener polarographischer Elektrode nach CLARK wurde der Sauerstoffverbrauch der jeweiligen Kultur ermittelt. Die Meßanordnung bestand aus einer Stabmeßzelle in Verbindung mit dem Sauerstoffmeßverstärker M65 F (VEB Meß- und Frequenztechnik Radebeul, DDR).

Bestimmung des pH-Wertes

Der pH-Wert wurde mit dem Präzisions-Labor-pH-Meßgerät MV88 (VEB PRÄCITRONIK Dresden, DDR) ermittelt.

Lactose-Bestimmung

Die Lactose-Bestimmung basierte auf der Methode von TELES u. a. [11]. Die dabei photometrisch zu messende Farbentwicklung beruht auf der kombinierten Wirkung von Phenol, NaOH, Pikrinsäure und Natriumhydrogensulfit mit Lactose. Gemessen wurde mittels „Spekol 10" bei 520 nm (VEB Carl Zeiss Jena, DDR).

Diacetyl-Bestimmung

Die Diacetyl-Bestimmung wurde nach der Methode von HETZEL [12] durchgeführt (o-Phenylendiamin-Methode). Die Messungen erfolgten mit Hilfe des Spektralphotometers VSU2 (VEB Carl Zeiss Jena, DDR) bei 335 nm.

Milchsäure

Die homofermentativ gebildete Milchsäure durch *Streptococcus cremoris* in rekonstituierter Magermilch (12.5 % Trockenmasse, Anfangs-pH-Wert 6,4) wurde anhand des gemessenen pH-Wertes über eine empirische Funktion nach JÖX et al. [13] errechnet:

$$x = \exp\left(\frac{y_{Me} - b}{a}\right) - c \tag{3}$$

x = Milchsäure [%],
y_{Me} = gemessener pH-Wert,
a = −1,67 (a, b durch Ausgleichsrechnung ermittelt)
b = 3,61
c = 0,18 (Modellkonstante).

Alle hier dargestellten Ergebnisse sind nur einige Beispiele aus umfangreichen Versuchsreihen. In jeweils mehreren identischen Versuchen konnte die Reproduzierbarkeit der Werte nachgewiesen werden.

Ergebnisse

1. Wachstumskinetik und Produktbildung der Reinkulturen

1.1. μ_{max} und K_s in Nährbouillon II

Wachstumskinetische Experimente erfordern für eine zuverlässige und nachvollziehbare Bestimmung von Zellkonzentration, Substraten sowie Produkten in der Kultur vor allem

standardisierte Nährlösungen. Nährbouillon II wird dieser Forderung gerecht. Im Gegensatz dazu bietet rekonstituierte Magermilch den Milchsäurebakterien ein optimales Milieu bezüglich ihres Wachstums, es bestehen jedoch erhebliche Schwierigkeiten für die Analytik zur Aufnahme von Wachstumskurven. Für die notwendige Abstufung der Substratkonzentration wäre außerdem als Ausgangsmedium eine sehr aufwendig herzustellende, lactosefreie Magermilch erforderlich.
Zur Bestimmung der kinetischen Parameter μ_{max} und K_s in Nährbouillon II wurde für die Aufnahme von Wachstumskurven bei 25 °C die Substratkonzentration im Bereich 0.05% bis 3% (unter sonst gleichen Milieubedingungen) variiert. Die Werte für μ_{max} und K_s wurden graphisch nach MONOD ermittelt (Abb. 1 u. 2), sie lauten:
L. citrovorum 1: $\mu_{max} = 0{,}55\ h^{-1}$, $K_s = 0{,}04$ g/l
L. citrovorum 78/80/L4/81: $\mu_{max} = 0{,}28\ h^{-1}$, $K_s = 2{,}0$ g/l
Sc. cremoris Scc_{77}/L4/81: $\mu_{max} = 0{,}35\ h^{-1}$, $K_s = 0{,}075$ g/l.

Sc. cremoris Scc_{77}/L4/81 zeigte zunächst ein stark vermindertes Wachstum in Nährbouillon. Erst durch Zugabe des Multivitaminpräparates „Summavit-flüssig" (VEB YSAT Wernigerode, DDR) konnte normales Wachstum erzielt werden.

Bei der Betrachtung der kinetischen Konstanten ist vor allem die hohe Variationsbreite zwischen den einzelnen Stämmen auffallend. Das hat besonders Konsequenzen für die Herstellung und den Praxiseinsatz von Starterkulturen (Mischkulturen), worauf in der Diskussion noch ausführlich eingegangen wird. Typisch für die MONOD-Kinetik ist die über einen weiten Bereich unabhängig von der Substratkonzentration gleichbleibende Wachstumsrate μ. Dieser Sachverhalt wird in Abb. 1 und 2 bestätigt. Substrathemmung trat bei diesen Konzentrationen nicht auf.

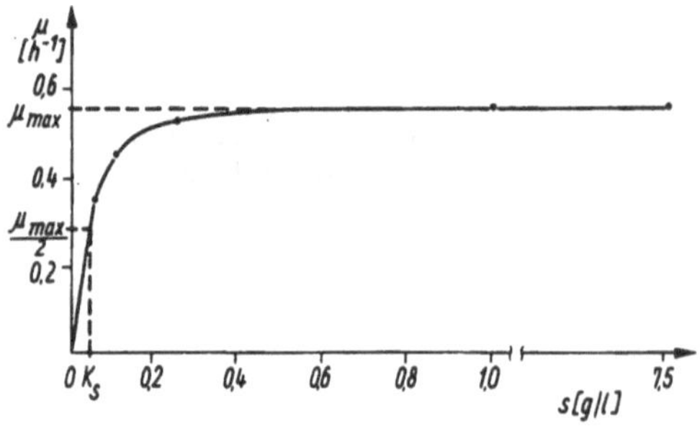

Abb. 1
Ermittlung von μ_{max} und K_s für *L. citrovorum 1* in Nährbouillon II, 25 °C, 4% Vorkultur. Die Kurve für μ nähert sich μ_{max} (gestrichelte Linie) asymptotisch

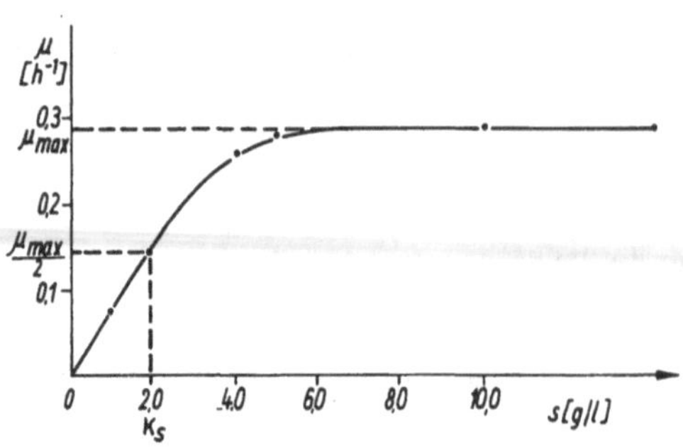

Abb. 2
Ermittlung von μ_{max} und K_s für *L. citrovorum* 78/80/L4/81 in Nährbouillon II, 25 °C, 4% Vorkultur. Zum Kurvenverlauf vgl. Abb. 1

1.2. Abhängigkeit des Wachstums von pH-Wert, Temperatur und Sauerstoff

pH-Wert

Beim Stamm *L. citrovorum* 78/80/L4/81 nahm die Wachstumsrate in Nährbouillon II in einer Versuchsreihe mit sinkendem pH-Wert zu Versuchsbeginn ab. Bei Anfangs-pH-Werten von 5,8 ... 6,0 wurden noch maximale Wachstumsraten erreicht (Abb. 3). Bereits bei pH-Wert 5,0 zu Beginn der Kultivierung betrug die Wachstumsrate nur noch 0,14 h^{-1}. Bei Wachstum in rekonstituierter Magermilch hatte die pH-Wert-Absenkung einen wesentlich geringeren Einfluß auf die Teilungs- bzw. Wachstumsrate für den o. g. Stamm (Tab. 1).

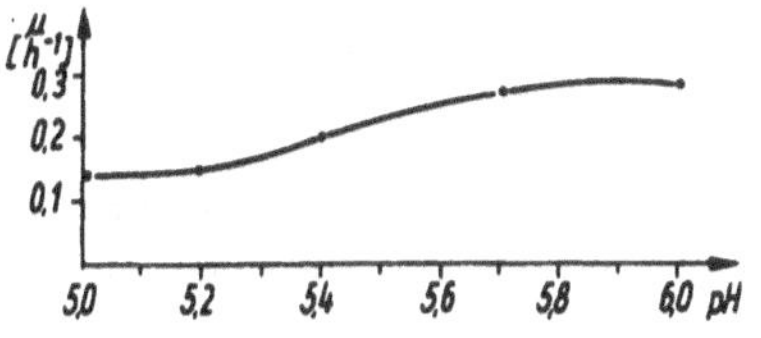

Abb. 3
Abhängigkeit des Wachstums von *L. citrovorum* 78/80/L4/81 vom pH-Wert zu Versuchsbeginn in Nährbouillon II, 25 °C

Tabelle 1
Einfluß des Anfangs-pH-Wertes in rekonstituierter Magermilch auf die Wachstumsparameter v und μ von *L. citrovorum* 78/80/L4/81

Anfangs-pH-Wert	Teilungsrate v [h^{-1}]	Spezifische Wachstumsrate μ [h^{-1}]
6,10	0,95	0,66
5,75	0,90	0,63
5,63	0,90	0,63
5,16	0,80	0,55

Temperatur

Für den Einsatz einer Starterkultur in der Praxis hat die minimale Wachstumstemperatur in den verschiedenen Rahmreifungsregimen besondere Bedeutung. Unter anderem auch deshalb wurde dem unteren Grenzbereich bei der Ermittlung der Temperaturabhängigkeit des Wachstums der Einzelstämme Beachtung geschenkt. Die Abhängigkeit des Wachstums von der Temperatur wurde für die Stämme *Sc. cremoris* Scc_{77}/L4/81 und *L. citrovorum* 78/80/L4/81 sowohl in Nährbouillon II als auch in rekonstituierter Magermilch ermittelt. Die Temperaturoptima liegen für den *Leuconostoc*-Stamm zwischen 25 ... 30 °C und für den *Streptococcus*-Stamm um 25 °C. Während *Leuconostoc* in Nährbouillon bei Temperaturen

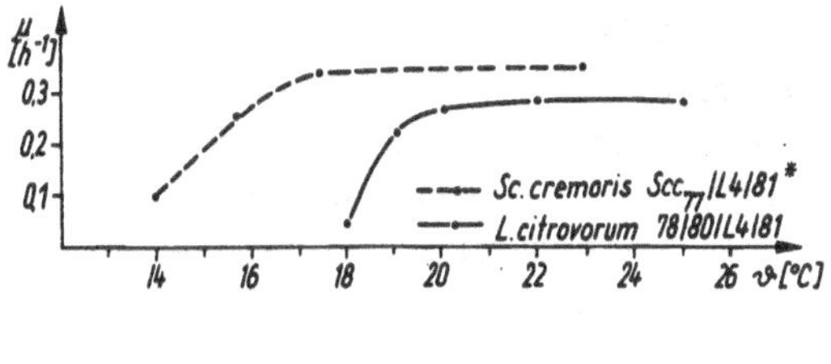

Abb. 4
Abhängigkeit des Wachstums von *L. citrovorum* 78/80/L4/81 und von *Sc. cremoris* Scc_{77}/L4/81 von der Temperatur in Nährbouillon II
* Wachstum Nährbouillon mit Vitaminzusatz

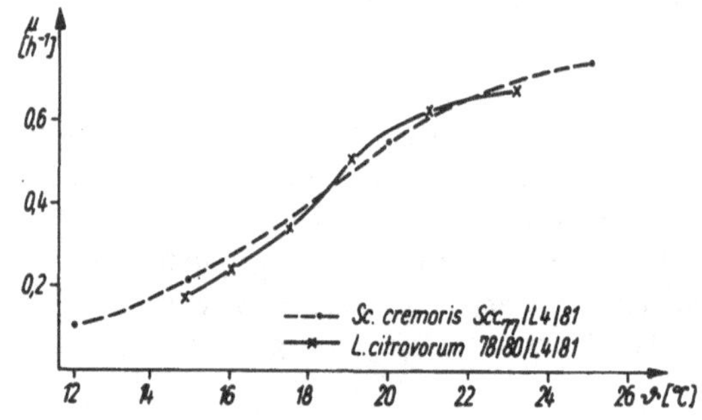

Abb. 5
Wachstum von *L. citrovorum* 78/80/L4/81 und von *Sc. cremoris* Scc_{77}/L4/81 in rekonstituierter Magermilch in Abhängigkeit von der Temperatur

unter 18 °C nicht mehr wuchs (Abb. 4), erreichte *Sc. cremoris* auch bei 16 °C noch Wachstumsraten um 0,28 h^{-1}, zeigte jedoch unter 14 °C kein Wachstum mehr. In rekonstituierter Magermilch dagegen trat für *Leuconostoc* erst unter 15 °C und für *Streptococcus* unter 12 °C Wachstumsstillstand ein (Abb. 5).

Sauerstoff

Der Einfluß der Sauerstoffzufuhr in Nährbouillon II auf das Wachstum erwies sich als stammspezifisch. Zusätzlicher Sauerstoffeintrag (durch Schütteln) bewirkte bei den hier untersuchten zwei *Leuconostoc*-Stämmen entweder nur geringfügige (Stamm 1) oder keine Erhöhung der Wachstumsrate. Ein von SCHNEIDER [14] untersuchter Stamm der Art *Leuconostoc citrovorum* erbrachte hingegen bei zusätzlichem Sauerstoffeintrag eine erheblich höhere Wachstumsrate (unter den gleichen Kultivierungsbedingungen). Von der Standkultur werden in 8 h maximal 3,2 mg O_2/l verbraucht.

In rekonstituierter Magermilch wurden für *L. citrovorum* 78/80/L4/81 bei der Schüttelkultur maximale Keimzahlen zwischen 12 und 15 h ermittelt, in der Standkultur lag dieser Bereich zwischen 14 und 16 h. Nach 24 h war bereits wieder eine Abnahme der Keimzahlen zu verzeichnen.

1.3. Substratabbau und Produktbildung

Nährbouillon II

Der Säuerungsverlauf führte bei Schüttel- und Standkulturen von *L. citrovorum* 1 zu ähnlichem Ergebnis. Der pH-Endwert ist vor allem von der Temperatur und darüber von der spezifischen Wachstumsrate abhängig. Mit steigender Temperatur in Richtung Wachstumsoptimum steigt auch die Produktsynthese. Bei *L. citrovorum* 78/80/L4/81 war mit sinkenden Anfangs-pH-Werten (unter pH 5,27) die Säuerungsleistung schwächer. Die Produktsynthese verringerte sich mit höherem Sauerstoffverbrauch ebenfalls.

Sowohl bei den heterofermentativen Leuconostoc-Stämmen als auch bei dem homofermentativen Lactatbildner *Sc. cremoris* Scc_{77}/L4/81 war in keinem Fall in der citratfreien Nährbouillon II die Aromakomponente Diacetyl nachweisbar. Die Lactose wurde nie vollständig abgebaut.

Rekonstituierte Magermilch

Alle in Magermilch durchgeführten Versuche sind als praxisnahe Untersuchungen zu verstehen. Zur Sicherung der konstanten Zusammensetzung der rekonstituierten Milch wurde nur sprühgetrocknetes Magermilchpulver einer einzigen Charge verwendet. Diese Magermilch hat eine Lactosekonzentration von 6,35 %.

Der nur schwach säuernde Stamm *L. citrovorum* 78/80/L4/81 erreichte nach 24 h pH-Werte um 6,0. Trotz Wachstumsstillstandes bei 14 °C konnte noch eine geringe Säuerung beobachtet werden. Bei einem pH-Wert von 6,1 produzierte dieser *Leuconostoc*-Stamm 0,04 mg Diacetyl/l, bei pH 5,4 (durch Zugabe von Milchsäure erreicht) bereits 3,5 ... 4,5 mg Diacetyl/l, was zu erwarten war. Das Maximum der Diacetylbildung lag bei 7 h, bereits nach 10 h erfolgte eine rasche Diacetylreduktion. Von der angebotenen hohen Lactosekonzentration der Magermilch wurden lediglich 3 ... 7 g/l verbraucht.

Sc. cremoris Scc_{77}/L4/81 hatte im Standkolben eine höhere Säurebildung als in der Schüttelkultur. Der Sauerstoffeintrag in der Schüttelkultur lag stets höher als der Verbrauch. Im Standkolben dagegen wurde der Sauerstoff fast vollständig abgebaut. Der Einfluß des Sauerstoffs auf den Substratverbrauch und die Milchsäurebildung bei Scc_{77}/L4/81 ist aus Tab. 2 ersichtlich. Bei Anwesenheit ausreichender Sauerstoffmengen wird wesentlich weniger Lactose verbraucht als bei Gärung unter mikroaerophilen Bedingungen. Der Produktbildungskoeffizient Y_S^P liegt bei der Schüttelkultur durchweg höher als bei der Standkultur, d. h. das Substrat wird unter Sauerstoffanwesenheit oxidativ und damit effektiver verwertet. So erreichte die Standkultur lediglich 50 ... 60 % der Substratverwertung der Schüttelkultur ($Y_{S\,K2}^P / Y_{S\,K1}^P$). Der Produktbildungskoeffizient ist stark temperaturabhängig; er hat bei 12 °C für *Sc. cremoris* Scc_{77}/L4/81 nur noch ein Drittel des Wertes von 25 °C (sowohl in Schüttel- als auch in Standkultur).

Für *Sc. cremoris* Scc_{77}/L4/81 war der Einfluß des Gelöstsauerstoffs auf das Wachstum wesentlich größer als bei den Leuconostoc-Stämmen. So wurde bei *Streptococcus* in fast allen Versuchen der Standkultur während der ersten 3 ... 4 h eine annähernd lineare Sauerstoffabnahme parallel zum Wachstum beobachtet (Abb. 6). Die Sauerstoffverbrauchsgeschwindigkeit ist ebenfalls temperatur- bzw. wachstumsabhängig. Bei 25 °C war der Sauer-

Tabelle 2
Einfluß von Sauerstoff und Temperatur auf Lactoseverbrauch, Milchsäurebildung und Produktbildungskoeffizient in Schüttel- und Standkultur von *Sc. cremoris* Scc_{77}/L4/81

Mikroorganismenart	Temperatur ϑ [°C]	Lactose-verbrauch S [g/l]		Milchsäure P_{gesamt} [g/l]		Produktbildungskoeffizient $Y_S^P \left[\frac{\text{g Milchsäure}}{\text{g Lactose}}\right]$	
		K_1	K_2	K_1	K_2	K_1	K_2
Sc. cremoris							
Scc_{77}/L4/81	25	3,4	20,01	1,44	5,22	0,425	0,261
	12	5,6	10,25	0,82	0,77	0,147	0,075

Nährmedium: Rekonstituierte Magermilch
K_1 = Schüttelkultur
K_2 = Standkultur

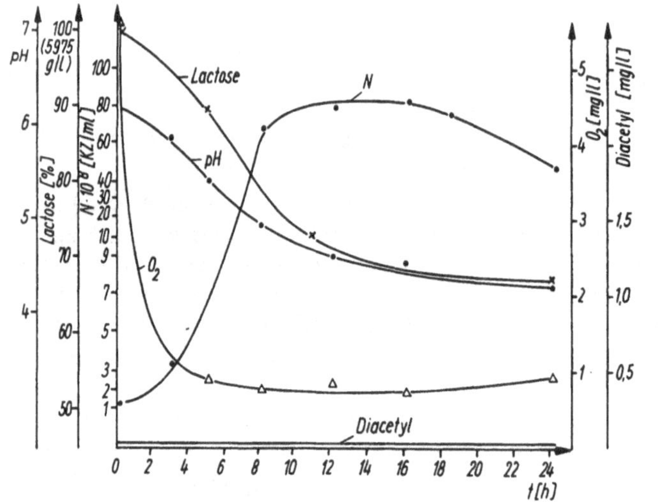

Abb. 6
Lactoseabbau, Säuerungsverlauf, Sauerstoffverbrauch, Diacetylnachweis und Wachstum von *Sc. cremoris* Scc_{77}/L4/81 in rekonstituierter Magermilch bei 25 °C, 4% Vorkultur

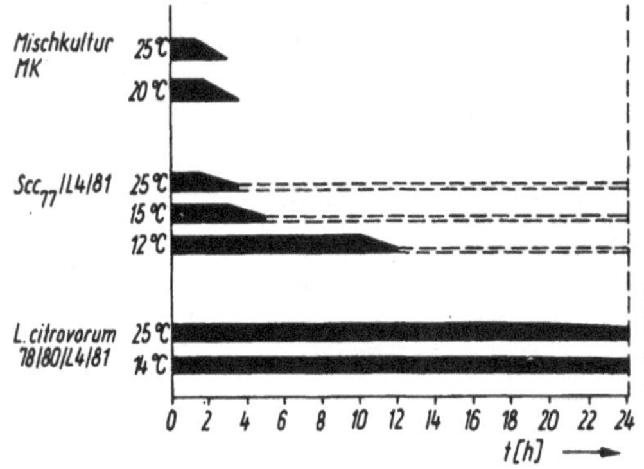

Abb. 7
Der Sauerstoffverbrauch in rekonstituierter Magermilch durch verschiedene Kulturen in Abhängigkeit von der Temperatur (4% Vorkultur)

stoff im Standkolben nach ca. 3 h und bei 15 °C erst nach 5 h verbraucht (Abb. 7). Scc_{77}/L4/81 produzierte in Magermilch und bei 25 °C kein Diacetyl, aber bei 12 °C konnten nach 24 h 0,3 mg/l nachgewiesen werden. Dieses Phänomen reiht sich in die Untersuchungsergebnisse von Thomas [15] ein, der in Starterkulturen eine Umschaltung von homofermentativer zu heterofermentativer Gärung bei limitierender Kohlenstoffquelle beobachtete. Es wird zudem als Hinweis betrachtet, daß die homofermentativen Lactatbildner auch die Enzymausstattung für heterofermentative Stoffwechselwege besitzen.

2. *Wachstum und Produktbildung ausgewählter Mischkulturen*

Da von allen handelsüblichen Starter-Mischkulturen lediglich die Mikroorganismenarten, jedoch nicht die Anzahl der entsprechenden Einzelstämme bekannt sind, ergeben sich Schwierigkeiten bei Untersuchungen von Populationsveränderungen und Syntheseleistungen der Mischkultur. Deshalb wurden zunächst Modell-Versuche mit einer genau definierten Zweistamm-Mischkultur (MK), bestehend aus 20% *L. citrovorum* 78/80/L4/81 und 80% *Sc. cremoris* Scc_{77}/L4/81, durchgeführt. Die Zusammenstellung der Mischkultur erfolgte erst jeweils kurz vor dem Einsatz; fortgezüchtet wurden beide Stämme als Einzelkultur. Die zweite getestete Mischkultur, die L-Kultur R23 (VEB WTÖZ der Milchindustrie der DDR, Oranienburg) diente als Vergleich.

2.1. μ_{max} *und* K_s *in Nährbouillon II*

Vorab muß darauf hingewiesen werden, daß die Bestimmung von μ_{max} und K_s bei Mischkulturen eigentlich nicht möglich ist, da diese Konstanten nur für Einzelstämme definiert sind. Die hierbei ermittelten Werte können deshalb lediglich zum Vergleich der Mischkulturen untereinander herangezogen werden. Die Kultivierung beider Mischkulturen in Nährbouillon war erst durch die Zugabe von Summavit (Multivitaminpräparat) möglich. Die Bestimmung von μ_{max} und K_s nach der Methode von Leineweaver/Burk ergab die Näherungswerte

Mischkultur MK: $\mu_{max} = 0{,}40\ h^{-1}$, $K_s = 0{,}36$ g/l
L-Kultur R23: $\mu_{max} = 0{,}35\ h^{-1}$, $K_s = 0{,}35$ g/l.

Wachstum in rekonstituierter Magermilch

In rekonstituierter Magermilch war das Wachstum beider Mischkulturen deutlich verbessert. Die Mischkultur MK erreichte hier μ-Werte um 0,85 h^{-1}, die L-Kultur R23 erzielte μ-Werte bis zu 1,0 h^{-1}.

2.2. *Substratabbau und Produktbildung*

Nährbouillon II

Beide Mischkulturen (MK und R23) sind gute Säurebildner. Sie säuerten innerhalb von 24 h bis zu pH 4,2 und verbrauchten dabei 4 ... 5 g Lactose/l. Bei Lactosekonzentrationen von 30 g/l ... 5 g/l wurde wesentlich mehr Milchsäure produziert als bei niedrigeren Lactose-Werten. Erst unter 0,7 ... 0,9 g Lactose/l wurde das Substrat vollständig abgebaut.

Der Sauerstoff war in Standkultur nach 2 ... 3 h fast vollständig aufgebraucht. Die Mischkulturen bildeten in Nährbouillon II kein Diacetyl.

Rekonstituierte Magermilch

Innerhalb 24 h sank der pH-Wert auf 4,5 ... 4,3 ab. In den Abb. 8 und 9 wird eine komplexe Darstellung des Zusammenhangs zwischen Wachstum, Substratverbrauch und Produktbildung aufgezeigt. Die Mischkultur MK erzielte maximale Diacetylwerte bis zu 10 mg/l. Die L-Kultur R23 war ein guter Diacetylbildner, es wurden Maximalwerte bis zu 18,5 mg/l erreicht. Es sei besonders darauf hingewiesen, daß die Diacetylbildung ihr Maximum nicht etwa nach 7 h (wie bei den Einzelstämmen von *Leuconostoc*) erreicht, sondern erst nach 12 ... 14 h (bei pH 5,0 ... 4,8). Bei optimalen Wachstumstemperaturen liegt die maximale Diacetylproduktion erst in der stationären Phase der Kultur vor. Bereits nach 16 ... 18 h war eine deutliche Reduzierung des Diacetyls zu verzeichnen.

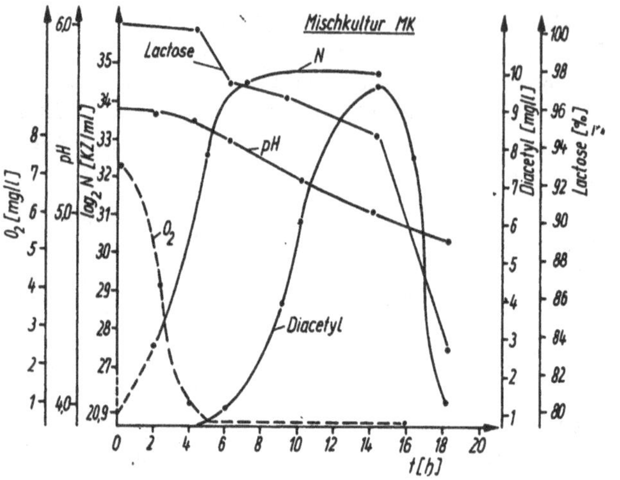

Abb. 8
Wachstum, Substratabbau und Produktbildung der Mischkultur MK in rekonstituierter Magermilch bei 25 °C, 4% Vorkultur

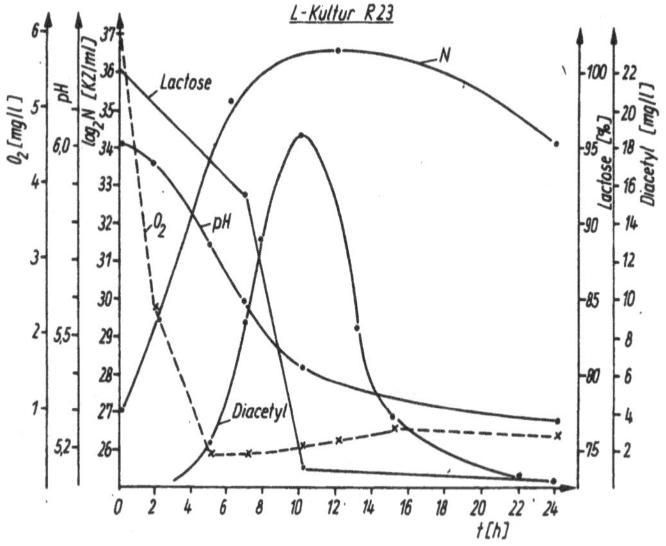

Abb. 9
Wachstum, Substratabbau und Produktbildung der L-Kultur R23 in rekonstituierter Magermilch bei 25 °C, 4% Vorkultur

Sowohl bei der Mischkultur MK als auch bei der L-Kultur R23 war in den ersten 4 h der Sauerstoff verbraucht.

2.3. *Überprüfung der Mischkultur MK im Praxiseinsatz eines Buttereibetriebes*

Obwohl die verwendeten Stämme *Sc. cremoris* Scc_{77}/L4/81 und *L. citrovorum* 78/80/L4/81 bezüglich ihrer Wachstumsparameter größere Unterschiede aufwiesen, erfolgte dennoch versuchsweise deren Praxiseinsatz, um u. a. folgerichtige Populationsveränderungen (Veränderung des Keimzahlverhältnisses Säurebildner/Aromabildner) bei solch ungünstiger Starterkulturenkombination nachzuweisen, die auch bei derzeit praktizierter Kombinationstechnik durchaus noch auftreten kann.

Fortzüchtung der Mischkultur MK als Betriebskultur

Für den Praxiseinsatz als Betriebskultur wurde die definierte Mischkultur MK in einem Buttereibetrieb in Rohmilch (1000 l Säureweckerbehälter) fortgezüchtet. Die Temperatur betrug 20 ... 21 °C (Tab. 3). Dabei säuerte die Kultur bis pH 4,13 und erreichte bei pH 4,20 eine maximale Diacetylproduktion von 2,19 mg/l. Besonders interessant ist hierbei, daß sich während der Fortzüchtung das Keimzahlverhältnis deutlich zugunsten von *Streptococcus*, nämlich von 1:4,5 bei 0 h bis 1:78 nach 17 h, änderte. Der Sauerstoffverbrauch entsprach dem in Magermilch.

Tabelle 3
Stoffwechselleistungen und Änderung des Keimzahlverhältnisses während der Fortzüchtung der definierten Mischkultur MK in 1000 l Rohmilch (2% Einsaatmenge)

Zeit t [h]	Temperatur ϑ [°C]	O_2-Abbau [mg/l]	Säuerung pH-Wert	Lactose-abbau S [g/l]	Diacetylbildung [mg/l]	Keimzahl-verhältnis L.c./Sc.c.
0	19	4,0	6,40	5,22	0,67	1:4,5
2,5	21	1,72	6,39	n. b.	0,53	1:6,7
4,5	21	n. b.	6,30	n. b.	0,53	1:37
10,5	21	0,52	5,26	4,18	0,81	1:20
13,5	21,5	n. b.	4,20	3,58	2,19	n. b.
17,5	21,5	0,34	4,13	3,28	2,00	1:78

n. b. = nicht bestimmt

Die Mischkultur MK im Rahmreifer

Nach 17 h Fortzüchtungsdauer kam die Mischkultur MK zum Betriebseinsatz der mikrobiologischen Rahmreifung. Es wurde das Kaltreifungsverfahren angewandt (Tab. 4). Im Rahmreifungstank traten Temperaturschwankungen von 11 bis 14,4 °C auf. Dieser Bereich entspricht der minimalen Wachstumstemperatur bzw. liegt geringfügig darunter (vgl. 1.2.). Deshalb wurden sowohl ein stark vermindertes Wachstum als auch eine verringerte Säuerungsleistung festgestellt. Der Sauerstoff war erst nach 12 h abgebaut und die Diacetylproduktion stieg bis 18 h nur allmählich an. Ein rascher Diacetylabbau war unter diesen Bedingungen jedoch nicht zu verzeichnen. Nach 23 h wurde ein pH-Wert des Rahms von 5,5 erreicht. Die Lactose wurde auch im Rahm nicht vollständig abgebaut. Die geringe Diacetylproduktion ist hauptsächlich auf das stark veränderte Keimzahlverhältnis während der Betriebskulturenherstellung zurückzuführen.

Diskussion

Die Bedeutung der Analyse zur Wachstumskinetik für den Kulturenhersteller und Anwender

Für eine effektive Einbeziehung der Wachstumsparameter μ_{max} und K_s wird deren naturwissenschaftliche Interpretation vorausgesetzt. Die Parameter μ_{max} und K_s sind genetisch determinierte Konstanten für jedes Stamm/Substrat-Paar. Bei Angaben von kinetischen

Tabelle 4
Stoffwechselleistungen und Wachstum der definierten Mischkultur MK während der Rahmreifung unter Produktionsbedingungen (2% Betriebskultur, 43% Rahmfettgehalt, 6000 l-Rahmreifungstank vom Typ ZRA)

Zeit t [h]	Temperatur ratur ϑ [°C]	O_2-Abbau [mg/l]	Säuerung pH-Wert	Lactose-abbau S [g/l]	Diacetyl-bildung [mg/l]	Keimzahl KZ × 10^7
0	11,0	8,46	6,61	2,68	0,34	4,2
2,5	13,2	8,39	6,60	n. b.	0,29	4,0
6,0	14,4	7,67	6,47	2,57	0,34	4,5
12,0	13,2	4,10	6,09	2,39	0,49	36
15	12,2	1,45	5,97	2,33	0,52	135
18	12,2	0,73	5,80 (5,5)*	2,21	0,57	n.b.
Butter aus gleichem Versuch					0,34	

n. b. = nicht bestimmt
* pH-Wert zur Verbutterung nach 23 h

Parametern sind deshalb stets die Kultivierungsbedingungen mit anzugeben, unter denen sie experimentell ermittelt wurden (Zusammensetzung des Nährmediums, Temperatur, pH-Wert . . .). Alle zu untersuchenden Stämme einer Mischkultur sind also unter identischen Bedingungen zu testen. Die Parameter μ_{max} und K_s liefern eine quantitative Aussage zum Wachstum des jeweiligen Mikroorganismenstammes. Nur durch quantitative Bewertungskriterien kann eine Stammauswahl bzw. eine Neukombination von Mikroorganismenstämmen eindeutig charakterisiert und optimiert werden. K_s sagt z. B. etwas über die physiologische Wachstumseffektivität aus. Kleinere K_s-Werte zeigen demnach Überlegenheit an gegenüber Stämmen mit größeren K_s-Werten, weil Stämme mit kleinen K_s-Werten schon hohe Wachstumsraten haben, wenn andere noch mit verringerter Geschwindigkeit oder gar nicht wachsen.

Aus dem Vergleich der Werte der untersuchten 2 *Leuconostoc*-Stämme und dem *Streptococcus*-Stamm für μ_{max}/K_s von 0,55 h^{-1}/0,040 g/l; 0,28 h^{-1}/2,0 g/l und 0,35 h^{-1}/0,075 g/l ist zu erkennen, daß diese Parameter offenbar in einem weiten Bereich liegen können. Diese großen Unterschiede sind oft Ursache für Populationsverschiebungen. Weiterhin ist zu beachten, daß die aromabildenden *Leuconostoc*-Stämme in einer Starter-Mischkultur zusammen mit den homofermentativen Lactatbildnern vorkommen. Ist in einer solchen Kultur ein *Leuconostoc*-Stamm mit einem großen μ_{max}- und einem geringen K_s-Wert vorhanden, so erfolgt in der Vorkultur eine viel stärkere Vermehrung der Aromabakterien. Daraus ergibt sich später eine Möglichkeit zur besseren Aromabildung [16]. Wenn sich aber im Gegensatz dazu ein Stamm mit einem geringeren μ_{max} und einem großen K_s in der Mischkultur befindet, wie z. B. der in den vorliegenden Untersuchungen verwendete Stamm *L. citrovorum* 78/80/L4/81, kann dessen Wachstum viel geringer sein. Dies hat eine Populationsverschiebung zugunsten der säurebildenden Streptokokken zur Folge (vgl. Tab. 3). Allgemein kann gesagt werden: Je größer die Differenz zwischen den μ_{max}-Werten ist, desto größer ist der Betrag in der Veränderung des Verhältnisses zwischen zwei Populationen. Dadurch ändert sich die Zusammensetzung der Starterkultur, und bei ihrem Einsatz ist eine optimale Rahmreifung nicht mehr gewährleistet. Weitere Faktoren wie Antagonismus und Phagenempfindlichkeit können in der gleichen Richtung wirken. Sie sind deshalb bei einer Stammkombination mit zu berücksichtigen.

Besonders für die Neukombination von Mischkulturen mit hoher Stabilität sind experimentelle Untersuchungen zur Wachstumskinetik von größter Bedeutung. Bezüglich einer Neukombination von Starter-Mischkulturen scheint es allgemein am günstigsten, wenn die Einzelstämme der Säure- und Aromabildner geringe K_s-Werte und große μ_{max}-Werte besitzen und diese Werte in ihrer Größenordnung übereinstimmen. In einem solchen Fall bestehen gleich gute Bedingungen für das Wachstum von Säure- und Aromabildnern. Stämme mit großem K_s-Wert haben außerdem eine geringere Säuerungsaktivität als solche mit kleinem K_s. Eine geringe Säuerungsaktivität bedeutet letztlich eine geringe Säurebildungsgeschwindigkeit. Dadurch wird der für die Diacetylbildung optimale pH-Wert erst später erreicht. Weiterhin begünstigt eine langsame Säuerung die Entwicklung von Fremdkeimen im Medium.

Das Wachstum einer Kultur wird u. a. von den Faktoren Substratkonzentration, Temperatur und pH-Wert beeinflußt. Die minimale Wachstumstemperatur ist dabei für den Starterkultureneinsatz gleichfalls von großer Bedeutung. Bei der Anzucht der Betriebskultur bei 19 ... 21 °C treten allgemein keine Probleme auf, da diese Temperaturen noch im Bereich der maximalen Wachstumsraten liegen. Aber das anschließend praktizierte Kaltreifungsverfahren für die Sauerrahmherstellung bewirkt bei Temperaturen von 10 ... 14 °C eine erhebliche Reduzierung des Wachstums. Hier kommt es zu weiteren Populationsverschiebungen, wenn starke Differenzen in der minimalen Wachstumstemperatur zwischen den einzelnen Stämmen vorhanden sind. Bei 12 °C war jedoch kein Wachstum bei den untersuchten Kulturen festzustellen. In diesem Fall kommt es offenbar vorwiegend über den Erhaltungsstoffwechsel zur Produktbildung.

Das Verhalten der Kulturen gegenüber Sauerstoff

Die beiden *Leuconostoc*-Stämme verhielten sich streng mikroaerophil, *Streptococcus cremoris* dagegen reagierte verstärkt auf den im Nährmedium angebotenen Gelöstsauerstoff (Abb. 7). So wurde in allen Versuchen (in der Standkultur) mit *Streptococcus* in Einzelkultur während der ersten 3 ... 4 h eine annähernd lineare Sauerstoffabnahme beobachtet (Abb. 6). Die logarithmische Wachstumsphase hielt jedoch nach dem Verbrauch des Sauerstoffs noch über weitere 4 h unvermindert an. WEINFURTNER et al. [17] machten ähnliche Beobachtungen mit *Lactobacillus pastorianus* und *E. coli*. Dieses Phänomen kann mit dem Umschalten von Teilatmung auf Vollgärung begründet werden. Bei den Mischkulturen MK und R23 belief sich die Zeit des unverminderten Wachstums auf ca. 2 h nach Erreichen der minimalen Sauerstoffkonzentration.

Durch den verstärkten oxydativen Abbau des Substrates bei Sauerstoffanreicherung im Nährmedium kommt es zur Hemmung der Milchsäurebildung (Tab. 2). Von den fakultativ anaeroben Mikroorganismen wird deshalb bei ausreichender Sauerstoffversorgung die Kohlenstoffquelle aerob abgebaut (Flavinatmung) und die freiwerdende Energie vorwiegend zum Aufbau neuer Zellsubstanz genutzt. In diesem Sinn kann der Sauerstoff als ein Steuerungsfaktor für die verstärkte Zellvermehrung während der Betriebskulturenherstellung betrachtet werden. Nach FORDYCE et al. [18] werden bei der aeroben Lactoseverwertung die gebildeten Pyruvat- und Lactatgehalte durch die entsprechenden Aktivitäten der NADH-Oxidase, NADH-Peroxidase und Lactatdehydrogenase bestimmt. Während des aeroben Wachstums von *Leuconostoc* ist Acetat ein Hauptendprodukt des Hexosemetabolismus [19].

Die Acetatsynthese über Acetatkinase benötigt kein energiereiches Phosphat. Dieses ist aber erforderlich, wenn Acetylphosphat zu Ethanol reduziert wird, um NAD^+ bei Abwesenheit von Sauerstoff zu regenerieren. Solch ein Mechanismus setzt ein O_2-abhängiges System der NADH-Oxidation voraus, um NAD^+ zu regenerieren. Das NAD^+ wird zur Dehydrierung von Glucose-6-phosphat und 6-Phosphogluconat benötigt. KAWAI et al. [20] und FITZGERALD [21] konnten solche NADH-Oxidasen in Leuconostoc-Stämmen nachweisen.

Die mikrobielle Produktbildung

In biotechnologischen Verfahren ist das primär angestrebte Ziel eine hohe Biomasse und/oder Produktbildung. Da das Wachstumsoptimum bei Starterkulturen nicht mit dem Optimum der Aromaproduktion übereinstimmt, ergibt sich die Aufgabe, das Wachstum der jeweiligen Population „produktorientiert" zu führen, um eine optimale Produktsynthese zu erhalten. Andererseits gilt für ein gutes Wachstum der Grundsatz: Je mehr Zellmasse vorhanden ist, um so mehr Produkt kann gebildet werden. Auch bei der mikrobiologischen Rahmreifung ist eine hohe Produktbildung (Säuerung, Aroma) das angestrebte Ziel. Bei der Rahmsäuerung handelt es sich um einen Spezialfall der Produktbildung, denn das Lactat wird aus dem energieliefernden Substrat Lactose gebildet. Dabei liegt ein wachstumsabhängiger und ein durch den Erhaltungsstoffwechsel gegebener wachstumsunabhängiger Substratverbrauch vor, die beide zur Produktbildung beitragen [22]. Im folgenden sollen einige wesentliche Faktoren zur Diacetylbildung zusammengefaßt werden: Das pH-Optimum zur Diacetylproduktion liegt zwischen 4,1 ... 5,5 und ist temperaturabhängig. Der optimale Zeitpunkt für das Diacetylmaximum ist ebenfalls von Temperatur und Stammzusammensetzung abhängig und liegt zwischen 12 und 18 h. Die optimale Temperatur für maximale Diacetylwerte liegt zwischen 14 und 16 °C, nachdem bei vorher höheren Temperaturen Wachstum, d. h. Vermehrung der Aromabildner erfolgte. Die Anwesenheit von Citronensäure (in rekonstituierter Magermilch originär in geringen Mengen vorhanden) ist eine grundlegende Voraussetzung für eine Diacetylproduktion, denn in citratfreier Nährbouillon der hier angestellten Versuche war in keinem Fall Diacetyl nachweisbar.

Offenbar ist die Diacetylbildung kein Vorgang des Primärstoffwechsels bzw. werden nur einige Reaktionsschritte davon benötigt. Über die entsprechenden peripheren Stoffwechselabläufe ist allgemein wenig bekannt. Bestimmte Empfehlungen zur Diacetylproduktion sind zwar besonders für die Praxis wichtig, tragen jedoch überwiegend zur Zeit noch phänomenologischen Charakter. Zumindest im Interesse einer hohen Aromaproduktion wäre es vorteilhaft, wenn vom Kulturenhersteller der Zeitpunkt für das zu erwartende Diacetylmaximum der gelieferten Kultur (z. B. bei Herstellung des Betriebssäureweckers oder bei Anwendung des Kaltreifungsverfahrens, mit Angabe standardisierter Kultivierungsbedingungen) dem Anwender mitgeteilt werden könnte. Dadurch bekäme der Anwenderbetrieb erstmals die Gelegenheit, sich bei Einhaltung der geforderten Prozeßparameter gezielt auf das zu erwartende Aromaoptimum einzurichten (Festlegung des günstigsten Zeitpunktes der Zugabe der Betriebskultur in den Rahmreifer bzw. des Verbutterungszeitpunktes).

Wachstum, Säuerung und Aromabildung einer Starterkultur müssen zwar differenziert, aber dennoch als Komplex gesehen werden. Die Analyse der einzelnen Abhängigkeiten scheint ohne eine bisher noch ausstehende Modellierung kaum möglich.

Summary

E. Jöx, A. Unger and H. Weide: Significance of growth kinetics and product formation for the selection and use of starter cultures in dairy industry

The activity of a starter culture (lactic acid and aroma production) is dependent on the stability of the combination of this mixed population and its optimal growth in the different periods of fermentation process. The growth parameters as specific growth rate (μ), maximum specific growth rate (μ_{max}), division rate (ν), doubling time (t_d), saturation constant (K_s) etc. of each single strain are the basis for the stability of a starter culture. Therefore the above mentioned parameters should be considered in production (novel combination) of starter cultures.

The growth kinetics of pure culture and mixed populations of selected lactic acid bacteria is examined and the significance of growth parameters μ_{max} and K_s of single strains for the production of starter cultures is discussed. The analysis of growth and product formation of single and mixed populations in reconstituted skim milk under consideration of environmental factors with practical relevance (pH, temperature, oxygen) offer possibilities of process control and optimization of product synthesis (lactic acid, diacetyl).

Резюме

Е. Йёкс, А. Унгер, Х. Вейде: Значение кинетики роста и образования продукта для выбора и использования заквасок в молочной промышленности

Активност закваски (продукция молочной кислоты и ароматических веществ) зависит от постоянства состава этой смешанной популяции и ее оптимального роста в различных фазах ферментативного процесса. Показатели роста специфический рост (μ), максимальная специфическая скорость роста (μ_{max}), скорость разделения (ν), время удвоения (t_d) и концентрация полунасыщения (K_s) каждого отделного штамма являются основой для стабильности закваски и поэтому их следует учитывать при производстве (новой комбинации) заквасок. Исследовалась кинетика роста чистых культур и смешанных популяций избранных молочнокислых бактерий и обсуждается значение показателей роста μ_{max} и K_s единичных штаммов для производства заквасок. Анализ роста и образования продукта единичных и смешанных популяций в реконституированном обезжиренном молоке с учетом важных для практики факторов окружающей среды (pH, температура, кислород) дает возможности для управления процессами и оптимизации синтеза продукта (молочная кислота, диацетил).

Literatur

[1] Sanders, M. E., P. J. Leonhard, W. D. Sing und T. R. Klaenhammer, Appl. environ. Microbiol. **52** (1986), 1001—1007.
[2] Klaenhammer, T. R., und R. B. Sanozky, J. gen. Mikrobiol. **131** (1985), 1531—1541.
[3] Mc Kay, L. L., und K. A. Baldwin, Appl. environ. Microbiol. **47** (1983), 68—74.
[4] Mc Kay, L. L., K. A. Baldwin und P. M. Walsh, Appl. environ. Microbiol. **40** (1980), 84—91.
[5] Jöx, E., Diss. A, Ingenieur-Hochschule Köthen, 1986.
[6] Sobeck-Skal, E., Inst. f. Mikrobiol., Hochschule f. Bodenkultur, 3—58, Wien 1961.
[7] Cogan, T. M., D. J. Buckley und S. Gondon, J. appl. Bacteriol. **34** (1971), 403—409.
[8] Collins, E. B., J. Dairy Sci. **60** (1977), 799—804.
[9] Cooper, R. K., und E. B. Collins, J. Dairy Sci. **61** (1978), 1085—1088.
[10] Kanasaki, M. u. a., Aust. J. Dairy Technol. **12** (1975), 142—152.
[11] Teles, F. F. F., K. C. Young und J. W. Stull, J. Dairy Sci. **61** (1978), 506—508.
[12] Hetzel, H. F., Milchwissenschaft **14** (1959), 424—429.
[13] Jöx, E., W. Pietzsch und M. Fröde, Lebensmittelindustrie **33** (1986), 79—80.
[14] Schneider, H., Dipl.-Arb., Ingenieur-Hochschule Köthen, 1980.
[15] Thomas, T. D., New Zealand J. Dairy Sci. Technol. **14** (1979), 12—15.
[16] Unger, A., Diss. A, Ingenieur-Hochschule Köthen, 1985.

[17] WEINFÜRTNER, F., A. UHL und H. OTT, Arch. Microbiol. **36** (1960), 1—22.
[18] FORDYCE, A. M., V. L. CROW und T. D. THOMAS, Appl. environ. Microbiol. (1984), 332—337.
[19] LUCEY, C. A., und S. CONDON, J. gen. Mikrobiol. **132** (1986), 1789—1796.
[20] KAWAI, K., S. YASHIMA, Y. OKAMI und Y. SASAKI, J. gen. appl. Mikrobiol. **17** (1971), 51—62.
[21] FITZGERALD, F. M., MSc thesis, University College, Cork, 1983.
[22] BERGTER, F., Wachstum von Mikroorganismen. Experimente und Modelle, Fischer, Jena 1983.

Dr.-Ing. E. Jöx, Prof. Dr. sc. H. WEIDE, Biotechnikum der Martin-Luther-Universität Halle-Wittenberg, Am Kirchtor 1, Halle, DDR-4020; Dr.-Ing. ANNEGRET UNGER, Institut für Impfstoffe Dessau-Tornau, Jahnstr. 8, Dessau, DDR-4500

Eingegangen 5. 5. 1987

Die Nahrung 32 (1988) 9, 855—859

Department of Food Chemistry, Toxicology and Applied Chemical Analysis,
Faculty of Pharmacy, University of Seville, Seville, Spain

Application of a new spectrophotometric method for Zinc determination in beverages and condiments

M. T. MORALES, M. T. MONTAÑA, G. GALÁN and J. L. GÓMEZ ARIZA

A new spectrophotometric method has been applied to the determination of zinc in bottled mineral water (with and without gas), refreshments, vinegar, and table salt. The method introduces the 1-[di-(2-pyridyl)-methylidene]-5-(salicylidene)-thiocarbohydrazone (DPST) as chromogenic reagent. This procedure is simple, rapid, reproducible and does not demand costly outfit and chemicals.

Introduction

Zinc is an essential element for humans. Minimum zinc requirements vary with age, functional activities, climatic conditions and the existence of stress imposed by trauma, parasitic infestation and infection [1, 2]. An important role for zinc on growth, keratogenesis, reproduction, skeletal development, wound healing, atherosclerosis, brain development and behaviour, protein and nucleic metabolism, carbohydrate and lipid metabolism, and enzyme activities in the tissues has been studied extensively [3]. So, it is very important to know the source and amount of zinc in oral intakes, and this has led to an increased interest in the determination of micronutrients in a wide variety of food products [4—11].

A survey of the literature reveals that a large number of reagents have been utilized for the spectrophotometric determination of zinc [12—14], but most of them lack adequate selectivity or they require liquid-liquid extraction. Dithizone [14] has been the most widely used for the absorptiometric determination of zinc in food [15—18], although the advantages and inconveniences of this non-selective, high sensitive reagent are also well known. For these reasons it was considered that a suitable method would be one that involved a direct measurement.

In this paper a new spectrophotometric method previously developed for us and applied to the determination of zinc in potable water [19] has been applied to the determination of this ion in bottled mineral water (with and without gas), refreshments, vinegar and table salt, in order to ascertain their contribution to the total intake through the diet.

The method is based on the interaction of zinc with 1-[di-(2-pyridyl)-methylidene]-5-(salicylidene)-thiocarbohydrazone (DPST) to form a yellow complex. The absorption spectrum indicates the formation of a single complex having its maximum at 417 nm, and the molar absorptivity was found to be $60500\ l \cdot mol^{-1} \cdot cm^{-1}$. The DPST — Zn complex is soluble in DMF-water, so the liquid-liquid extraction is not necessary.

Materials and methods

The content of zinc was determined in 5 samples of vinegar, 5 of table salt, 10 of bottled mineral water (5 with gas and 5 without), and 5 of refreshments, by the DPST method and AAS for comparison.

Apparatus

Absorption spectra and absorbances were measured with Bausch and Lomb Spectronic 2000 spectrophotometer. Quartz cells (1.00 cm path length) were used throughout the work.

A Beckman model 70 and Crison model 501 pHmeters with combined saturated calomel glass electrodes were used for pH measurements. Throughout this paper pH is used to denote pH-meter reading and not actual concentration of hydrogen ions in solution.

Atomic-absorption measurements were carried out using Perkin-Elmer model 2380 instrument.

Reagents

Reagent solutions were prepared from analytical-reagent grade chemicals and were dissolved in deionized water.

The 1-[di-(2-pyridyl)-methylidene]-5-(salicylidene)-thiocarbohydrazone (DPST) was prepared as described previously [19]. A 0.1 % (v/v) solution in dimethylformamide was prepared; this solution was stable for several months.

Standard zinc solution, 5.2060 $g \cdot l^{-1}$. Prepared by dissolving the appropiate amount of zinc sulphate pentahydrate in distilled water and standardizing titrimetrically with EDTA using murexide as indicator. Working solutions were prepared by suitable dilution.

Buffer solution (pH 5.3). Prepared by dissolving 13.4 g of sodium acetate trihydrate and 2.1 ml of acetic acid conc. in water and diluting to one litre.

Procedure

Pipette suitable aliquots containing up to 25 µg of zinc into 25 ml calibrated flasks. Add 2.5 ml of DPST solution and 5 ml of dimethylformamide, mix and add 5 ml of buffer solution. Dilute the solution to the mark with deionized water and mix well. Measure the absorbance at 417 nm against a reagent blank. The calibration graph was prepared from standard solution of Zn(II) treated in the same way.

Results and discussion

As we have indicated in a previous paper [19] zinc ions react with DPST in weakly acidic medium (pH 5.3) to form a yellow complex having maximum absorbance at 417 nm. The complex was formed immediately and the absorbance remained constant for 24 h.

BEER's law is obeyed between 0.0 and 1.0 ppm. The linear regression equation obtained by a least-squares treatment is $A = 9.26 \times 10^{-1} |Zn| + 1.4 \times 10^{-2}$ ($r = 0.999$). The molar absorptivity calculated from the above equation was $6.05 \times 10^4 \; l \cdot mol^{-1} \cdot cm^{-1}$. The optimum concentration range, evaluated by RINGBOM's method, was 0.21—0.94 ppm. The relative standard deviation for 0.31 ppm of zinc ($n = 11$, $p = 0.05$) was $\pm 0.81\%$. For the investigation of between-day variations, single determinations were made on different days. All the absorbances were within the range 0.288—0.310 (0.31 ppm of zinc) and the relative standard deviation was $\pm 1.54\%$.

The effect of diverse species on the determination of zinc has also been investigated. Good results were obtained on masking Cu(II), Bi(III), Hg(II) and Pb(II) with thiosulphate, and

Table 1
Zinc content in vinegar

Sample no.	Volume taken [ml]	Zinc found [ppm ± s.d.]*	Masking agent citrate [ppm]	Zinc found by AAS [ppm]
1	1.0	3.02 ± 0.02	5000	2.99
2	0.5	5.75 ± 0.05	5000	5.72
3	1.0	0.87 ± 0.04	4500	0.88
4	2.0	0.59 ± 0.01	6500	0.60
5	2.0	0.52 ± 0.03	5000	0.51

* Mean of three determinations.

Table 2
Zinc content in table salt

Sample no.	Amount taken [g/100 ml]	Volume taken [ml]	Zinc found [ppm ± s.d.]*	Masking agent citrate [ppm]	Zinc found by AAS [ppm]
1	5.000	10	0.061 ± 0.003	—	0.06
2	5.000	10	0.070 ± 0.009	3000	0.08
3	5.000	10	0.075 ± 0.005	3000	0.08
4	5.000	10	0.070 ± 0.008	—	0.08
5	5.000	10	0.036 ± 0.006	3000	0.03

* Mean of three determinations.

Table 3
Results of zinc recovery from beverages

Sample	No. of samples	Zn(II) added [μg]	Zn(II) found [μg ± s.d.]*	Recovery [%]
Bottled mineral water with gas	5	0	—	
		5	5 ± 0.04	100
		10	10 ± 0.05	100
		20	20 ± 0.02	100
Bottled mineral water without gas	5	0	—	
		5	5 ± 0.05	100
		10	10 ± 0.03	100
		20	20 ± 0.03	100
Refreshments	5	0	—	
		5	5 ± 0.03	100
		10	10 ± 0.03	100
		20	20 ± 0.02	100

* Mean of three determinations.

Fe(II), Fe(III) and Ni(II) with citrate. Thiosemicarbazide and iodide masked the interferences due to small amounts of Co(II) and Cd(II).

Determination of zinc in condiments

Because of the simplicity of the direct DPST procedure, its applicability to the determination of microgram amounts of zinc in vinegar and table salt was studied, and the results are compiled in Tables 1 and 2. The interference caused by the presence of iron in some samples was eliminated by addition of citrate as masking agent. The results were in good agreement with those obtained by atomic absorption spectrometry and from these it can be deduced that these condiments are an important source of Zn(II) in the diet of the Spanish population.

Determination of zinc in beverages

The zinc content in bottled mineral water (with and without gas) and refreshments was investigated. To check the accuracy of the method the samples were spiked with different concentrations of zinc as zinc(II) sulphate and analyzed as already described. Unspiked samples were also investigated by atomic absorption spectrometry. The results shown in Table 3 are in good agreement with the expected values.

Conclusions

The DPST method has been shown to be applicable to the determination of zinc in condiments and beverages. The method is simple, sensitive and rapid. It is labour-saving and less sensitive to light than the dithizone method. The few interferences encountered can be eliminated by simple masking; its main disadvantage is that it requires meticulous cleanliness in order to prevent contamination.

Zusammenfassung

M. T. Morales, M. T. Montaña, G. Galán und J. L. Gómez Ariza: Anwendung einer neuen spektrophotometrischen Methode zur Zinkbestimmung in Getränken und Würzmitteln

Es wurde eine neue spektrophotometrische Methode zur Bestimmung von Zink in abgefülltem Mineralwasser (mit und ohne Gas), Erfrischungsgetränken und Tafelsalz angewendet. Bei dieser Methode dient 1-[Di-(2-pyridyl)-methylen]-5-(salicyliden)-thiocarbohydrazon (DPST) als chromogenes Reagenz. Das Verfahren ist einfach, rasch durchführbar, reproduzierbar und benötigt keine kostspieligen Apparaturen und Chemikalien.

Резюме

М. Т. Моралес, М. Т. Монтана, Г. Галан, и Й. Л. Гомез Ариза: Применение нового спектрофотометрического метода для определения цинка в напитках и специях

Для определения цинка в расфасованной минеральной воде (с газом и без газа), освежающих напитках и повареной соли исползовался новый спектрофотометрический метод. При этом методе хромогенным реактивом служит I-[ди-(2-пиридил)-метилен]-5-(салицилиден)-тиокарбогидразон (DPST). Способ простой, быстры воспройзводимый и не требует больших затратов для оборудования и химических реактивов.

References

[1] Halsted, J. A., J. C. Smith and M. I. Irwin, J. Nutr. **104** (1974) 345.
[2] Sandstead, H. H., Curr. Top. Nutr. Dis. **6** (1982) 83.
[3] Underwood, E. J., Trace Elements in Human and Animal Nutrition, 4. ed, p. 196. Academic Press, London 1977.
[4] Reith, J. F., J. Enjetsma and M. van Ditmarsch, Z. Lebensm.-Unters. Forsch. **156** (1974) 271.
[5] Lindner-Szotyori, K., and L. Eutropia, Elelmiszervizsgalati Kozl, **20** (1974) 329.
[6] Crithrie, B. E., N. Z. Med. J. **82** (1975) 418.
[7] Piekacz, H., Zesz. Probl. Postepow Nauk Roln. **179** (1976) 485.
[8] Allen, K. G. D., and L. M. Klevag, Nutr. Rep. Inst. **16** (1977) 227.
[9] Lindner-Szotyori, K., and A. Gergely, Nahrung, **24** (1980) 829.
[10] Welsh, S. O., and R. M. Marston, Food Technol. **36** (1982) 70.
[11] Barberá, R., and R. Farré, Nahrung **30** (1986) 565.
[12] Sandell, E. B., Colorimetric Determination of Trace Metals, 3. ed. Interscience, New York 1959.
[13] Fries, J., and H. Getrost, Organic reagent for Trace Analysis. Merck, Darmstadt 1977.
[14] Marcenko, Z., Spectrophotometric Determination of Elements. Ellis Horwood, Westergate, England, 1976.
[15] Stone, I., Wallerstein Lab. Commun. **25** (1962) 329.
[16] Balogh, G., and E. Felszeghy, Studia Univ. Babes-Bolyai, Ser. Chem., **12** (1967) 97.
[17] Parkash, S., and R. Jenness, J. Dirg Sci. **50** (1967) 127.
[18] Khrisanfova, L. P., and B. G. Rostortsev, Dokl. TSKHA, **157** (1970) 117.
[19] Morales, M. T., M. T. Montaña, G. Galán and J. L. Gómez Ariza, Analyst **112** (1987) (in press).

M. T. Morales, Dr. M. T. Montaña, G. Galán and J. L. Gómez Ariza, Department of Food Chemistry, Toxicology and Applied Chemical Analysis, Faculty of Pharmacy, University of Seville, 41012 Seville, Spain

Received May 6, 1987

Rezensionen

Protein Tailoring for Food and Medical Uses. Herausgegeben von R. E. Feeney und J. R. Whitaker. 392 Seiten, zahlr. Abb. und Tab. Marcel Dekker, Inc., New York und Basel 1986.

„Maßgeschneiderte Proteine", vielstrapaziertes Schlagwort aus dem Bereich der Lebensmittelchemie, wird hier in einem sehr allgemeinen Sinne für solche Proteine gebraucht, die durch zielgerichtete Veränderung ihrer Struktur ganz bestimmte Eigenschaften erlangt haben, so daß sie entweder paßgerecht als funktioneller Bestandteil in Lebensmittelsystemen, als lebensmitteltechnologisch relevante Enzyme oder aber als biologisch spezifisch wirkende Proteine im medizinischen Sektor einsetzbar sind. Die 14 Beiträge des vorliegenden Buches, hervorgegangen aus Vorträgen eines gleichnamigen Symposiums der American Chemical Society, berücksichtigen unterschiedliche Aspekte der Modifizierung von Proteinen durch chemische, enzymatische und gentechnische Manipulationen bzw. zielgerichtete Wechselwirkung.

Der einführende Artikel (R. E. Feeney: Tailoring Proteins for Food and Medical Uses: State of the Art and Interrelationships) faßt den aktuellen Kenntnisstand zusammen. Die chemische Modifizierung von Nahrungsproteinen wird in Arbeiten über die kovalente Verknüpfung essentieller Aminosäuren mit Proteinen zur Verbesserung der ernährungsphysiologischen und funktionellen Eigenschaften (J. R. Whitaker) und über die Verknüpfung stark hydrophober Aminosäureester mit nativem oder enzymatisch abgebautem Protein zur Erzielung von Proteinen mit besonderer Oberflächenaktivität oder Gefrierschutz-Eigenschaft (S. Arai, M. Watanabe, N. Hirao) abgehandelt. Zwei Beiträge zum Komplex der enzymatischen Modifizierung betreffen das Problem der sensorischen Eigenschaften von Proteinhydrolysaten (J. Adler-Nissen: Relationship of Structure to Taste of Peptides and Peptide Mixtures) und die Erzeugung biologisch aktiver Peptide aus Proteinen am Beispiel opiater Peptide aus Milchproteinen (H. Chiba, M. Yoshikawa). Weitere Beiträge behandeln die Prinzipien und Anwendungsmöglichkeiten des Genetic Engineering für Enzyme und Nahrungsproteine (R. Jimenez-Flores, Y. C. Kang, Th. Richardson) sowie deren spezielle Anwendung im medizinischen Bereich (R. Wetzel), ferner das Problem der Modifizierung von Proteinen über spezifische Wechselwirkungen am Beispiel der Suizid-Inaktivatoren (R. B. Silverman: Mechanism-based Enzyme Inactivation for Medical Uses), der Affinitätsreagentien für Enzyme (W. F. Benisek, M. Hearne: Probing the Active Site of a Steroide Isomerase with a Solid Phase Reagent) und der Wechselwirkung von Proteintoxinen mit der Zelloberfläche (K. Sandvig, S. Olsness).

Die Erzeugung spezifischer biologischer Wirkungen durch chemische Modifizierung ist Gegenstand von 4 Beiträgen, in denen die Kupplung mit Antikörpern im Hinblick auf die Zellspezifität von Proteintoxinen (J. W. Marsh, D. M. Neville), Albumin-Enzym-Konjugate als vielseitige Therapeutika (M. J. Poznansky), Bindungen von Metallionen an Antikörper mittels bifunktioneller Chelatreagentien (Cl. F. Meares) sowie die maßgeschneiderte Synthese eines Antitumorproteins durch Kupplung mit einem Polystyren-maleinsäureanhydrid-Copolymeren (H. Maeda, Y. Matsumura, T. Oda, K. Sasamoto) beschrieben werden.

Die Vielfalt der Themen dieses Bandes spiegelt eine Tendenz internationaler Nahrungsprotein-Symposien wider, Funktionalität von Proteinen über den lebensmitteltechnologischen Aspekt hinaus auch in ihrer ursprünglichen biologischen Bedeutung zu erfassen. Die jüngste Entwicklung der Proteinchemie zeigt deutliche Übergänge zwischen beiden. Die Gewinnung biologisch aktiver Peptide aus Nahrungsproteinen beweist, daß diese mehr darstellen als nur Aminosäurequellen für die Eiweißneusynthese. Die vorliegende Publikation ist bestens geeignet, zu einer entsprechend universelleren Betrachtung der Reaktionen und Wechselwirkungen von Proteinen anzuregen und darüber hinaus auch Betrachtungen über den Sinn und die Grenzen des Genetic Engineering von Nahrungsproteinen anzustellen.

K. D. Schwenke

Vertebrate Cell Culture I. Herausgegeben von A. Fiechtner. 166 Seiten, 39 Abb., 28 Tab. Akademie-Verlag, Berlin 1987. Preis: 118,— M.

In den letzten Jahren hat die Kultivierung von Säugetierzellen im Zusammenhang mit der Untersuchung von Zellfunktionen, aber auch als Basis für biotechnologische Produkte eine immense Bedeutung erlangt. Für den letzten Fall stellt die Ablösung eines serumsubstituierten durch ein definiertes serumfreies Kulturmedium den entscheidenden Durchbruch gegenüber Produkten konventioneller Verfahren dar. In insgesamt 8 Übersichtsreferaten wird die schrittweise Einführung von serumfreiem Kulturmedium bei der Kultivierung von verschiedenen Zelltypen sowie bei der Produktion von Tollwut- und MKS-vakzinen beschrieben.

D. W. R. Bleyl

Die Nahrung 32 (1988) 9, 861—865

Prague Institute of Chemical Technology, Department of Food Chemistry, Prague, Czechoslovakia

Residues of clopyralide (3,6-dichloropicolinic acid) in strawberries and their changes

JANA HAJŠLOVÁ, ZUZANA JEHLIČKOVÁ, F. PUDIL and J. DAVÍDEK

Residues of clopyralide in strawberries treated with herbicide preparation Lontrel 300 were determined using gas chromatographic method. The decrease of clopyralide content during the processing of contaminated fruits was observed. The rate of decomposition of this compound in model solutions (held at 75 °C, pH 3,6) followed first-order kinetics. 2,5-dichloropyridine was proved to originate under these conditions from parent compound.

Introduction

Clopyralide (3,6-dichloropicolinic acid) is an active ingredient of Lontrel 300 manufactured by Dow Chemical Co. This potent foliar-applied growth-regular herbicides is intended for phenoxy-tolerant weed control, especially in cereals, rape and sugar beets [1]. Clopyralide was introduced as a substitute of other chemically related herbicide — picloram (4-amino-3,5,6-trichloropicolinic acid) displaying high persistency in soils and crops [2—4]. Based on the results of some field trials [1], half-life of clopyralide was assessed to be approximately a quarter of that observed for picloram. Following treatment, clopyralide is easily translocated throughout the plant. The rate of residues dissipation in sugar beets was studied in a detail [5, 6].

The aim of this study was to follow the fate of clopyralide residues in strawberries both under field conditions and during the processing of contaminated fruit.

Materials and methods

Materials

Strawberries (Senga Sengana) were treated with Lontrel 300 at a dose 0.3; 0.4; 0.8 kg/ha before the blooming of the plants. Field experiments were carried out in the years 1985 and 1986. The interval between the treatment and analysis of matured fruit is given in Table 1.

Chemicals

Clopyralide (3,6-dichloropicolinic acid, Dowco 290) was supplied in the 99.3 % purity by Dow Chemical CO. (England). Diazald (p-tolylsulphonylmethylnitrosamide) was used for the preparation of diazomethane [7]. All other chemicals were of reagent grade.

Procedure

Similar procedure as that recommended by GALOUX et al. [6] for analysis of sugar beets was used for isolation and derivatization of clopyralide residues: 50 g of strawberries were homogenized in 150 ml of 0.25 M potassium hydroxide. The homogenate was filtered through the Celite 545 layer on a Büchner funnel. This filter was rinsed with 50 ml of hydroxide solution and two 50 ml portions of water. Combined filtrates were acidified by 70 ml 4 M sulphuric acid and after the addition of 30 g sodium chloride, the extraction of residues was carried out by two portions (150 ml and 50 ml) of diethyl ether. The combined extracts were dried over anhydrous sodium sulphate and then evaporated under vacuum (the temperature of the water bath held at 40 °C) up to dryness. 7 ml of diazomethane solution (in diethyl ether) were used for the esterification of clopyralide residues, an excess of derivatizing agent was removed (after 4 h) by a gentle stream of nitrogen. The volume of the sample was adjusted up to 3 ml by diethyl ether, aliquots were used for gas chromatographic analyses.

In stability studies, model solutions containing 1 mg of clopyralide in 50 ml of citrate buffer (pH 3.6) were held at 75 °C. The same procedure as described above was used for clopyralide determination starting with extraction of acidified aqueous reaction mixtures (pH 2) by diethyl ether. In the case of 2,5-dichloropyridine determination, pH value of model solutions was adjusted to 5 prior to the diethyl ether extraction step. No methylation of this compound was necessary for gas chromatographic analysis.

Gas chromatography

Gas chromatograph Hewlett Packard 5880 A equipped with ^{63}Ni EC detector and terminal integrator unit (level four) was used for analyses. Chromatographic separations were carried out on 2400 mm × 2 mm (i.d.) glass column with 10% Carbowax 20 M (on Chromaton N-AW-DMCS, 0.125—0.160 mm) operated under the following conditions: oven temperature 200 °C, flow rate of carrier gas (nitrogen) 30 ml/min. Temperature of injection port was 230 °C, that of detector 300 °C.

Mass spectrometry

Mass spectra (ionization voltage 70 eV) were recorded (after gas chromatographic separation) by Jeol DX 300 (Japan) instrument.

Results and discussion

Good separation of clopyralide methylester from other volatile compounds co-isolated from strawberries was achieved using column packed with Carbowax 20M (Fig. 1). Retention time of our analyte was under the conditions used 7.4 min; an increase of the oven temperature up to 220 °C (for approx. 5 min) can be recommended after elution in order to achieve quicker cleaning of the column.

The mean value of recovery in the range 0.01—2.0 mg of clopyralide per 1 kg of spiked strawberries was (90.2 ± 0.8)%, the lowest detectable amount of this herbicide was 0.005 mg/kg. In Table 1, the residue values determined in strawberries treated with various doses of Lontrel 300 are given. As expected, successive decrease of residues occurred during the harvest period. It is obvious, that the residue levels correspond to the amount of applied herbicide preparation, surprising proportionality was manifested in experiment B—D carried out in the same year and in the same locality. The total content of residues, however, depended on the climatic conditions that occurred both in the course of fruit growing and harvesting. Relatively high levels of clopyralide contained in strawberries at the beginning of the harvest period in experiment A were probably due to minor rainfall in preceding

Table 1
The content of clopyralide in matured strawberries treated with Lontrel 300

Experiment*	Dose of Lontrel 300 [kg/ha]	Residues of clopyralide [mg/kg]** Days after application:	
		45	58
A	0.3	0.380	0.098
B	0.3	0.056	0.048
C	0.4	0.079	0.069
D	0.8	0.150	0.130

* A — performed in the year 1985, B—D in the year 1986
** Average value obtained from 4 parallel determinations

weeks. Intensive rainwashing of leaves and leaching of the herbicide from the surface layers of the soil can be assumed to have contributed to the significant decrease of residues in following rainy days.

As strawberries are widely used for the preparation of various heat-processed products including fruit baby food, the stability of clopyralide under similar conditions was investi-

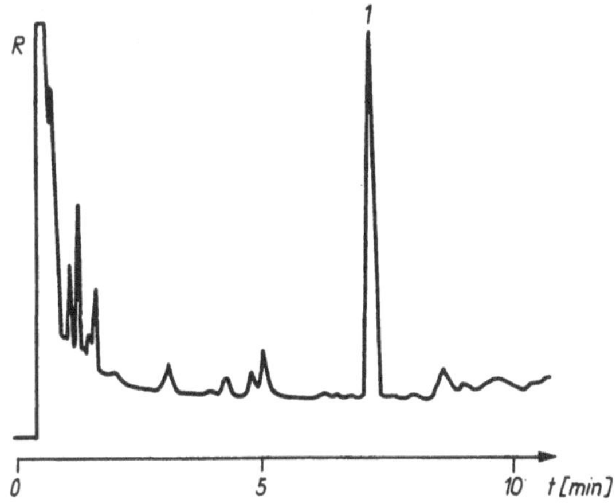

Fig. 1
Gas chromatographic determination of clopyralide in contaminated strawberries. The injection represents the equivalent of 50 mg of sample (0.1 mg of clopyralide per kg was added).
1 — peak corresponding to methylester of clopyralide.

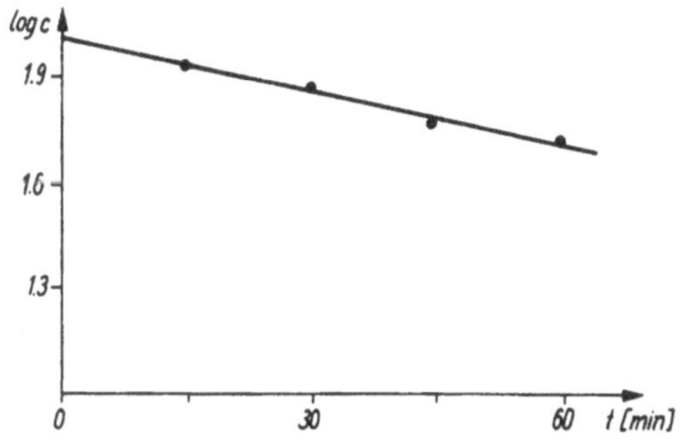

Fig. 2
The degradation of clopyralide in buffered aqueous solution (pH 3.6, temperature held at 75 °C).
c — concentration of clopyralide [%]

gated in our further experiments. Only 68.2% of initial clopyralide content (0.1 mg/kg) was determined in spiked strawberries homogenate heated 30 min at 75 °C.

The decrease of clopyralide amount in citrate buffer (pH 3.6 — i.e. the same value as that of juice from strawberries) heated at 75 °C is shown graphically in Fig. 2. Based on the values obtained, degradation of this compound proceeded according to the first-order kinetics. The first-order rate constant under these conditions was calculated to be $1.98 \cdot 10^{-4}$ s^{-1}. Having determined clopyralide in heated model solutions, we observed the presence of a new volatile compound at retention time 1.7 min (none was contained in unheated samples). By means of coupled gas chromatography — mass spectrometry 2,5-dichloropyridine was identified in this chromatographic zone. Mass spectra of both 2,5-dichloropyridine and methylester of clopyralide are shown in Fig. 3. At higher mass region the same base ions can be seen at m/z 147 (being identical with molecular peak for 2,5-dichloropyridine). They would be suitable for simultaneous mass-fragmentographic (single ion monitoring) determination of both analytes. It is conceivable that 2,5-dichloropyridine will arise via decarboxylation of 3,6-dichloropicolinic acid. In order to achieve maximum yield of 2,5-dichloropyridine, pH value of aqueous solution should be adjusted to at least 5 prior to the extraction by diethyl ether. According to the basic nature of pyridine, one would expect higher pH value to be necessary, however, chlorine atoms (displaying negative induction effect) substituting a heterocyclic ring can be assumed to be responsible for the decrease of basicity. Good stability of 2,5-dichloropyridine in the course of methylation procedure (used for volatilization of 3,6-dichloropicolinic acid) was proved, no origination of new volatile compounds and/or a decrease of analyte peak were observed. The presence of 2,5-dichloropyridine in heat sterilized strawberries was revealed, too. Supposing com-

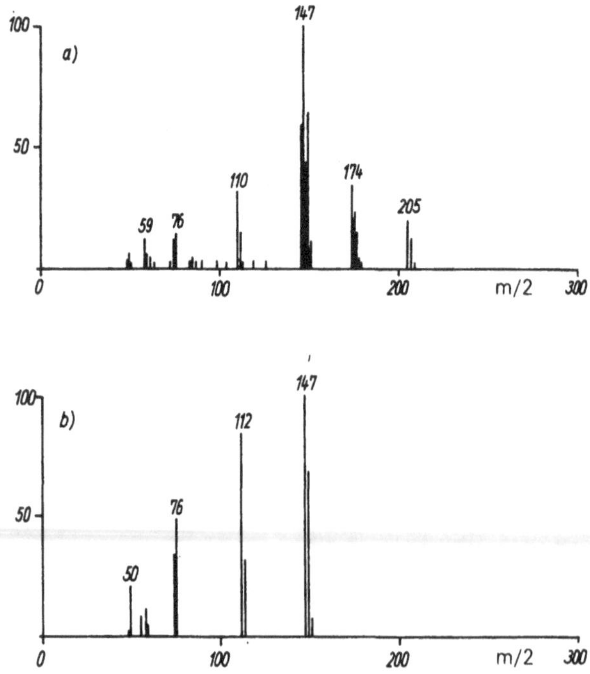

Fig. 3
Mass spectra of methylester of clopyralide (a) and 2,5-dichloropyridine (b).

parable ECD response for both 2,5-dichloropyridine (its standard was not available) and clopyralide methylester, approximately 5 μg/kg of chlorinated pyridine discussed were determined in spiked homogenate (0.1 mg of clopyralide per 1 kg of strawberries) after heating for 30 min at 75 °C. In case that only 2,5-dichloropyridine gas chromatographic determination is intended, the column temperature should be held lower — e.g. at 150 °C (retention time of analyte 4.7 min) as it enables better separation of this relatively more volatile substance (in comparison with clopyralide methylester) from other compounds contained in analyzed extracts.

Based on all the recognized facts, it can be concluded, that despite a decrease of clopyralide residues as the result of heat sterilization procedure, the origination of other compounds suspectable from the hygienic point of view should be taken into account.

Zusammenfassung

J. HAJŠLOVÁ, Z. JEHLIČKOVÁ, F. PUDIL und J. DAVÍDEK: Rückstände von Clopyralide (3,6-Dichlorpicolinsäure) in Erdbeeren und ihre Veränderungen

Clopyralide (der Wirkstoff des Herbicides Lontrel 300) wurde in den damit behandelten Erdbeeren gaschromatographisch ermittelt. Während der Verarbeitung der kontaminierten Früchte nahm der Gehalt an Clopyralide ab. Der Abbau dieser Verbindung in Modellösungen (Temperatur 75 °C, pH 3,5) verlief nach einer Reaktion erster Ordnung. Es konnte nachgewiesen werden, daß unter diesen Bedingungen aus der Ausgangssubstanz 2,5-Dichlorpyridin entsteht.

Резюме

Й. ХАЙСЛОВА, З. ЕГЛИЧКОВА, Ф. ПУДИЛ и И. ДАВИДЕК: Остаточные количества клопиралида (3,6 дихлоропиколиновой кислоты) в клубнике и их изменения

С помощью газовой хроматографии исследовались остатки клопиралида в клубнике после аппликации гербицида Лонтрел 300. Во время переработки загразненных плодов наблюдалось снижение содержания клопиралида. Скорость разложения в моделных растворах при температуре 75 градусов и pH 3,6 соответствовала кинетике первого порядка. Оказалось, что в таких условиях возникает 2,5 дихлоропиридин.

References

[1] Dow Chemical Co., Technical Information on Dowco 290, Midland, Mich., 1974.
[2] Picloram: The effects of its use as herbicide on environmental quality, National Research Council of Canada, Publication NRCC No. 13684, p. 17, 1974.
[3] BAUR, J. R., R. D. BAKER, R. W. BOVEY and J. D. SMITH, Weed Sci. **20**, 305 (1972).
[4] REDEMANN, C. T., R. W. MEIKLE, P. HAMILTON, V. S. BANKS and C. R. YOUNGSON, Bull. Environ. Contam. Toxicol. **3**, 80 (1968).
[5] GALOUX, M. P., J. C. VAN DAMME and A. C. BARNES, J. Chromatogr. **242**, 323 (1982).
[6] GALOUX, M. P., J. C. VAN DAMME, A. C. BARNES and J. F. SALEMBIER, J. Agric. Food Chem. **31**, 759 (1983).
[7] VOGEL, A. I., Practical Organic Chemistry, p. 20. Longmans, London 1961.

Ing. JANA HAJŠLOVÁ, CSc., Prague Institute of Chemical Technology, Department of Food Chemistry, CS-166 28 Prague 6 — Dejvice, Suchbátarova 1905, Czechoslovakia

Received May 20, 1987

Rezensionen

Topics in Lipid Research. From structural elucidation to biological function. Herausgegeben von R. KLEIN und B. SCHMITZ. 336 Seiten, zahlr. Abb. und Tab. The Royal Society of Chemistry, London 1986. Preis: 37,50 £; 65,— $

Die Monographie basiert auf den Beiträgen und Diskussionen des Symposiums „Beziehungen zwischen Struktur und Funktion der Lipidmoleküle und deren makromolekular geordneter Systeme", das die Royal Society of Chemistry im April 1986 in Cambridge, UK, veranstaltete und an dem überwiegend westeuropäische Wissenschaftler teilnahmen. Die Herausgeber versuchen dabei eine Synthese zwischen Übersichtsarbeiten und speziellen Forschungsberichten, um den modernen Wissensstand möglichst umfassend aus biophysikalischer, biochemischer, physiologischer und pharmakologischer Sicht darzustellen.

Die Sektion „Plättchenaktivierungsfaktor" umfaßt Chemie und Physiologie der Glyceroglycolipide, die u. a. bei der Blutgerinnung eine Rolle spielen, sowie deren Antagonisten und die Regulation ihrer Biosynthese. In der Sektion „Eicosanoide" stehen die Prostaglandinendoperoxide, Thromboxane und Prostacycline im Mittelpunkt, wobei auch analytische Fragen behandelt werden. Den verschiedensten Glycolipiden der Bakterien ist die recht ausführliche Sektion 3 gewidmet, besonders orientiert auf deren Isolierung, Analyse und Strukturaufklärung. Die Sektion „Membranstruktur und Funktion" stellt die gegenwärtigen Forschungstrends zur Analytik, Modifikation und Funktionscharakterisierung biologischer Membranen heraus, die Sektion „Umweltadaptation" beleuchtet u. a. die Rolle der Bakterienmembranlipide bei der phylogenetischen Entwicklung, die Thermodynamik bei der Adaptation sowie die Temperatur- und Druckabhängigkeit des Membrantransports. Die Round-table-Diskussion zur Problematik des Einflusses von Probenentnahme und der Anästhetika auf die Untersuchungsergebnisse und Schlußfolgerungen rundet das sehr anspruchsvolle, mit zahlreichen Literaturangaben versehene Werk ab. Es wird in erster Linie dem Spezialisten vorbehalten bleiben, die Übersichtsbeiträge könnten aber auch für einen breiteren Leserkreis von Interesse sein.

L. AUST

The Impact of Chemistry on Biotechnology (ACS-Symposium Series 362). Developed from a symposium sponsored by the Biotechnology Secretariat at the 192nd Meeting of the American Chemical Society, Anaheim, California, September 7—12, 1986. Herausgegeben von M. PHILLIPS, S. P. SHOEMAKER, R. D. MIDDLEKAUFF und R. M. OTTENBRITE. 415 Seiten, zahlr. Abb. und Tab. American Chemical Society, Washington, DC, 1988. Preis: 95,95 $ (USA und Canada 79,95 $).

Einleitend werden die historische Entwicklung der Biotechnologie sowie der Anteil der Chemie daran dargestellt und Trends aufgezeigt. CAD-Lösungen für biochemische Prozesse, die anaerobe Umwandlung von Cellulose (auf Rohstoffbasis fester Siedlungsabfälle) zu C2-, C3- und C4-Carbonsäuren, das Scale-up von Trennverfahren (hohes mathematisches Niveau des Beitrages) und die Warmblüterzelltechnik (mit deren Umsetzung in Bioreaktoren und Kostenanalysen in Varianten) stellen jeweils gesonderte Kapitel vor. 4 Beiträge über Polymere in der Medizin (Anstieg des Marktes 1985 zu 1990 um das 2- bis 3fache wird prognostiziert) berichten über polymere Arzneimittel, polymere Träger für Wirkstoffe, an Polymere gebundene Konjugate sowie Applikationssysteme, Liposomenmembranen aus polymeren Lipiden und Proteine sowie Peptide in Verbindung mit medizinischen Fragestellungen (Glycosyltransfer, Kontaminationen mit DNA und Pyrogenen, Synthesen u. a.). Die zwei Artikel über analytische Sachverhalte betrachten Konformationsanalysen bei Proteinen sowie den Nachweis von Kontaminanten in Proteinen, die mittels rDNA-Techniken gewonnen wurden. Im Komplex Agrochemie werden die Anwendungen von *Bacillus thuringiensis*, Immunoassays für Pestizide (Harnstoffderivate u. a.), enzymatische Verfahren zur Pheromonsynthese sowie die mikrobielle Gewinnung von Avermectin (ein Antiparasitikum) betrachtet.

6 Artikel sind dem Gebiet landwirtschaftlicher Rohstoffe/Lebensmittel gewidmet, wobei allgemeine Trends aufgezeigt werden und speziell die symbiotische Stickstoff-Fixierung, die Photosynthese-Regulierung und die Pflanzenzüchtung berücksichtigt wurden. Den Abschluß der informativen Monographie bilden Beiträge zum Marketing (Biotechnologiemarkt: Stand, Trend; Beispiele für Verfahren: Vitamin C, Acrylamid, Phenylalanin, Diagnostika) sowie zur Versorgung mit Informationen auf dem Fachgebiet. Darin enthalten werden Teilaspekte zur Risikobeurteilung moderner Biotechnologie angesprochen. Die Monographie weist eine gelungene Mischung von allgemeine Aspekte berührende und spezielle Sachverhalte vorstellende Beiträgen auf.

R. MACHOLZ

Die Nahrung **32** (1988) 9, 867—873

Technical University Budapest, Department of Biochemistry and
Food Technology, Budapest, Hungary, and Agricultural Biochemistry Department, Faculty of Agriculture,
El Minia University, El Minia, Egypt

Biochemical studies of some non conventional sources of protein. Part 4. The proteins of mango waste stone kernels[1]

R. Lásztity, M. A. El Shafei, M. B. Abdel Samei, F. S. Hatour and M. Labib

The gross chemical composition, protein content and amino acid composition of mango stone kernels of four Egyptian varieties (Ewsi, Hendi, Fonso and Timour) were investigated. Carbohydrates are the main components of the seed. The protein content varies between 5.0 and 7.2% and the ether extract ranged from 10.8% to 13.6%. High glutamic acid, aspartic acid and leucine content and low concentration of sulfur-containing amino acids are characteristic for the proteins of mango kernels. Lysine level is also low, the concentration of other essential amino acids is acceptable. Sulfur-containing amino acids are the first limiting ones followed by lysine and threonine.

Egypt imported for the first time, in 1825, budded trees of mango from Bombay which established themselves successfully. Since then, this fruit has been growing well there, and now it covers an area of 3233 ha, mostly in Lower and Middle Egypt. Most of the Egyptian varieties are of Indian origin [1].

Production, however, is small relative to the size of the population in Egypt and there is a definite need for a large-scale expansion of the crop. Mango is cultivated in Egypt in about 9% of the total area under fruit cultivation. According to the latest official report over 67770 tons of mangoes are produced annually in this area. Depending upon variety and size, 30 to 50% of the fruit are waste in the form of peels and stones, which could be probably profitably utilized for the preparation of some important and useful by-products. The utilization of this waste would not only solve the problem of its disposal but would also reduce the price of processed mango products.

The mango is the second tropical fruit (banana occupies the first place) in terms of production and area of cultivation, and it is one of the important fruit crops of the world. Convenience foods, including processed products and fruit beverages based on mango have gained importance in recent years over the world. So it is understandable that a growing number of publications related to the investigation of mango appears in the scientific journals.

Review papers resp. books of Jain [2], Singh [3], Hulme [4] and Subramanyan et al. [5] give a general information about the growing, storage and composition of mango. The problem of the food value of mango stone kernels is also discussed in some papers [6—9]. Utilization of mango stone kernels is also treated in some publications [5, 10—12]. According to these publications the seeds are comparable to most of the cereals, particularly in respect to carbohydrate, fat, protein, minerals, calcium and phosphorous. Relatively few

[1] Part 3 Nahrung **30** (1986) 629

data are available concerning the variations in protein content, the amino acid composition and nutritional quality of the proteins.

In this paper an attempt has been made to evaluate some of the possible by-products that can be prepared from local mango stone kernels. We hope that will be an incentive for initiating planned research and investigation into the problem of processing of mango stone kernels. Some of the aspects worth looking into are: Chemical composition of the kernels, scopes for proper and effective utilization of the by-products and more over the biological value of its proteins. Such study would be highly valuable in harnessing the enormous amount of this raw material which, at present, entirely goes waste and thus providing probably a new non-conventional protein source.

Material and methods

Samples

Four local varieties of Mango Fruits (*Mangifera indica* L.) variety Ewsi, Hendi, Fonso and Timour were collected from the fruit research station, Dokki, Giza, Egypt. After weighing the fruit, skin and pulp were removed. Freshly depulped mango stones were collected and washed in a current of water to free them from adhering pulp, fiber, dirt etc. The washed stones were air-dried. Stone and kernel were separated and weighed.

Chemical analysis

The chemical composition (moisture, total nitrogen, lipid, ash and fiber) of duplicate samples was determined according to the standard methods of Association of Official Agriculture Chemists [13]. The protein content of each sample was calculated by multiplying the nitrogen content by the conversion factor 6.25. The total sugars, expressed as glucose, were determined quantitatively as described by Dubois et al. [14].

Mineral analysis

The minerals were determined colorimetrically, flamephotometrically and with atomic-absorption spectrophotometry (Perkin-Elmer model 303). The analyses were carried out in the laboratory for soil and plant testing, Soil Science Department, Minia University.

Amino-acid analysis

The amino acid composition was analysed on an automatic amino acid analyzer (Beckman, Model 121). The tryptophan content was determined colorimetrically as described by Blauth et al. [15]. The amino acid scores were determined referring to the provisional amino acid scoring pattern of the Food Agriculture Organization and the World Health Organization [16].

Results and discussions

Mango stone of different four local varieties: Ewsi, Hendi, Fonso, and Timour, were found to be always consisted of a tenacious leathery outercoat and an inner kernel. The kernels in the stone amount to about 62—79% of the mango seeds. No relationship was

Table 1
Chemical composition and mineral contents of Mango kernels of four local varieties (dry weight basis)

Mango kernel varieties	Moisture [%]	Crude fibre [%]	Ash [%]	Ether extract [%]	Crude protein [%]	Carbohydrate* and undermined materials [%]	P [%]	K [%]	Na [%]	Mn [ppm]	Zn [ppm]	Fe [ppm]
Ewsi	11.7	2.5	2.2	13.6	5.03	65.0	0.02	0.75	0.73	22.0	15.0	60.0
Hendi	11.3	2.1	2.0	11.8	5.77	67.1	0.04	0.85	0.63	9.0	12.0	—
Fonso	10.7	2.5	2.4	11.5	5.94	67.1	0.01	1.66	0.95	24.0	16.0	74.0
Timour	10.3	2.2	2.7	10.9	7.19	66.8	0.02	1.56	0.85	29.7	18.4	86.5

* Calculated by difference

Table 2
Total amino acids of defatted mango kernels (expressed as g/16 g N)

Amino acids	Mango kernel varieties			
	Ewsi	Hendi	Fonso	Timour
Essential amino acids				
Isoleucine	3.24	3.38	3.11	2.82
Leucine	8.30	9.42	10.0	10.74
Histidine	5.57	5.63	5.63	6.41
Lysine	1.13	1.82	1.75	1.77
Methionine	0.08	0.30	0.06	0.08
Phenylalanine	3.14	2.58	2.22	2.56
Threonine	1.53	2.58	2.10	2.27
Valine	5.82	6.70	5.99	6.31
Tyrosine	1.09	0.78	1.05	1.14
Tryptophan	0.80	0.90	0.90	0.90
Cystine	0.30	0.24	0.11	0.26
Non essential amino acids				
Alanine	2.94	2.67	2.03	2.19
Arginine	4.19	0.64	3.33	3.43
Aspartic acid	14.2	15.0	14.0	13.2
Glutamic acid	27.5	28.6	25.2	24.7
Glycine	5.35	5.30	5.37	5.30
Proline	4.35	5.41	4.22	3.82
Serine	0.95	1.51	1.41	1.48
Total amino acids	89.4	97.4	88.5	89.2
Total essential amino acids	31.0	34.3	32.9	35.1
Total nonessential amino acids	58.4	59.1	55.6	54.0,
E/T ratio [%]	34.7	36.8	37.8	39.3

found between fruit weight and seed content; but the higher the fruit weight the lower the kernel content.

The average values of the chemical composition of the kernels of the four local mango varieties are shown in Table 1.

The protein content varies from 5.0% to 7.2%. The ether extract ranges from 10.8% to 13.6%. Hendi variety was found to contain the lowest level of crude fiber (2.1%) whilst Timour was found to contain the highest percentage of ash content (2.7%) when compared to other varieties. Our results agree with those reported by other authors [2, 5, 10—12].

The total amino-acid composition of the four local varieties of mango kernels are reported (Table 2, 3). Results are expressed as percentage of 16 g N as well as dry matter, respectively. The results indicated that the two dicarboxylic amino acids aspartic acid and glutamic acid, in all different varieties represented the highest crude protein percentage when compared to other amino acids analysed. No other acid could compete with the acidic amino acids except the leucines (Table 2).

Among all amino acids determined in all varieties, the lowest percentage was those of sulphur-containing amino acids and tryptophan.

As far as differences of amino acids percentage among varieties are concerned, the data reveal that such differences do exist, and may be attributed to interspecific variations.

According to FAO/WHO [16] the total amino acid proportion (E/T ratio) that must be supplied as essential amino acid is suggested to be 36% of the protein amino acids composition.

In all examined varieties the essential amino acids averaged from 31.0 to 39.4%, thus showing a relatively good E/T ratio (Table 2).

Deficiencies of sulphur-containing amino acids were reflected in their respective scores of 10.9; 15.4; 4.9 and 9.7 for Ewsi, Hendi, Fonso and Timour varieties, respectively. The

Table 3
Essential amino acids content of the four local variety of Mango kernels*

Amino Acids	Mango kernel varieties			
	Ewsi	Hendi	Fonso	Timour
Leucine + isoleucine	0.90	0.99	1.03	1.27
Lysine	0.08	0.14	0.14	0.17
Total sulphur amino acids	0.029	0.042	0.014	0.032
Cystine	0.023	0.019	0.009	0.024
Methionine	0.006	0.023	0.005	0.008
Total aromatic amino acids	0.30	0.26	0.26	0.35
Phenylalanine	0.22	0.20	0.18	0.24
Tyrosine	0.08	0.06	0.08	0.11
Threonine	0.11	0.20	0.17	0.21
Tryptophan	0.06	0.07	0.07	0.08
Valine	0.45	0.52	0.47	0.59

* Expressed as % of dry defatted matter [g/100 g]

Table 4
Essential amino acid content (EAA) and amino acid score of Mango kernel seeds and the FAO/WHO provisional scoring pattern

Amino acid	Mango kernel varieties								
	Ewsi		Hendi		Fonse		Timour		FAO/WHO [16]
	EAA [g/16 g N]	Amino acid score	EAA [g/16 g N]	Amino acid score	EAA [g/16 g N]	Amino acid score	EAA [g/16 g N]	Amino acid score	EAA [g/16 g N]
Leucine + Isoleucine	11.5	104.9	12.8	116.4	13.1	119.4	13.6	123.3	11.0
Lysine	1.13	20.6	1.82	33.1	1.75	31.8	1.77	32.2	5.5
Total sulphur amino acid	0.38	10.9	0.54	15.4	0.17	4.86	0.34	9.7	3.5
Cystine	0.30		0.24		0.11		0.08		
Methionine	0.08		0.30		0.86		0.26		
Total aromatic amino acid	3.23	70.5	3.36	56.0	3.27	54.5	3.7	61.7	6.0
Phenylalanine	3.14		2.58		2.22		2.56		
Tyrosine	1.09		0.78		1.05		1.14		
Threonine	1.53	38.3	2.58	64.5	2.1	52.5	2.27	56.8	4.0
Tryptophan	0.8	80.0	0.9	90.0	0.9	90.0	0.8	80.0	1.0
Valine	5.82	116.4	6.7	134.0	5.99	119.8	6.31	126.2	5.0

second limiting amino acid was lysine. Threonine was the third limiting amino acid, whilst the total aromatic amino acids were the fourth ones (Table 4).

It is worthy to note that mango kernels alone are a nutritionally poor protein source due to low amounts of methionine and cystine. Nevertheless it seems that the high amount of some other essential amino acids give a possibility to produce mixtures of good nutritional value which should be useful in countries cultivating enormous amounts of this fruit.

An incorporation of methionine by enzymatic modification as used in other proteins [17] may be also possible. Elaboration of some optimal mixtures and a more complex evaluation concerning the biological value and availability of amino acids based on own and other experiments [18—20] will be included in the further research work.

Zusammenfassung

R. LÁSZTITY, M. A. EL SHAFEI, M. B. ABDEL SAMEI, F. S. HATOUR und M. LABIB: Biochemische Untersuchungen über einige nicht konventionelle Proteinquellen. 4. Mitt. Die Proteine der Kerne von Abfall-Mangosteinen

Die chemische Zusammensetzung der Makrobestandteile, der Eiweißgehalt und die Aminosäuren-Zusammensetzung der Kerne von Mangosteinen von vier egyptischen Sorten (Ewsi, Hendi, Fonso und Timour) wurde untersucht. Kohlenhydrate sind die Hauptbestandteile der Samen. Der Eiweißgehalt liegt zwischen 5,0 und 7,2%, die Menge des Etherextraktes beträgt 10,8% bis 13,6%. Hohe Glutaminsäure-, Asparaginsäure- und Leucingehalte und niedrige Konzentration an schwefelhaltigen Aminosäuren sind charakteristisch für die Mangosamen. Die Lysin-Konzentration ist ebenfalls niedrig; die Menge der anderen essentiellen Aminosäuren ist ausreichend. Schwefelhaltige Aminosäuren sind die ersten limitierenden Aminosäuren vor Lysin und Threonin.

Резюме

Р. ЛАСТИТЫ, М. А. ЭЛЬ-ШАФЕЙ, М. Б. АБДЕЛЬ САМЕЙ, Ф. С. ХАТОУР и М. ЛАБИБ: Биохимические исследования некоторых нетрадиционных источников белка. Сообщ. 4. Белки ядер отбросок косточки манго

Исследовались химический состав макрочастей, содержание белка и аминокислотный состав ядер косточек манго четырех египетских сортов (Ewsi, Hendi, Fonso, Timour). Основными сотавными частями семян являются углеводы. Содержание белка составляет от 5,0 до 7,2%, количество эфирного экстракта равняется 10,8% до 13,6%. Характерными для семян манго является высокое содержание глютаминовой кислоты, аспарагиновой кислоты и лейцина и низкая концентрация серосодержащих аминокислот. Концентрация лизина также низка; количество остальных незаменимых аминокислот достаточное. Серосодержащие аминокислоты являются первыми лимитирующими аминокислотами перед лизином и треонином.

References

[1] EL-TOMI, A. L., Proc. Fla. Hort. Soc. **66** (1953) 195—201.
[2] JAIN, N. L., Rev. Food Technol. **3** (1961) 131—162.
[3] SINGH, L. B., The Mango. Leonhard Hill, London 1960.
[4] HULME, A. C., in: The Biochemistry of fruits and their products. Ed. by A. C. HULME. Vol. 2, p. 233 to 240. Academic Press, New York 1971.

[5] SUBRAMANYAM, H., S. KRISHNAMURTHY and H. A. B. PORPIA, Food Res. **21** (1975) 223—305.
[6] DAS, N. B., Food value of Mango-seed kernel. Food Council Publication, New Delhi 1971.
[7] KEHAR, N. D., and R. CHANDA, Curr. Sci. **15** (1946) 48—50.
[8] EL-SHAFEI, M. A., M. B. ABDEL SAMEI and R. LÁSZTITY, Minia J. Agr. Res. and Dev. **8** (1986) 417—426.
[9] LAKSHMINARAYANA, G., T. CHANDRASEKHARA RAO and P. A. RAMALINGASWAMY, J. am. Oil Chem. Soc. **60** (1983) 88—89.
[10] IKRANUL HAG, M. Y., and A. F. M. EHTESHAMUDDIN, Sci. Ind. **8** (1971) 207—209.
[11] ABDEL SAMEI, M. B., R. LÁSZTITY and M. A. EL-SHAFEI, Minia J. Agr. Res. and Dev. **8** (1986) 429—447.
[12] NARASIMHA CHAR, B. L., B. R. REDDY and S. D. THIRUMALA RAO, J. am. Oil Chem. Soc. **54** (1977), 494—495.
[13] Official Methods of Analysis of the Association of Official Analytical Chemists (AOAC). Ed. by W. HORWITZ, 12th ed. AOAC, Washington, DC, 1975.
[14] DUBOIS, M., K. A. GILLES, J. K. HAMILTON, P. A. REBERS and F. SMITH, Anal. Chem. **28** (1956) 350 — 356.
[15] BLAUTH, O. J., M. CHARAINSKI and H. BERBEE, Anal. Biochem. **8** (1973) 69—73.
[16] FAO/WHO, Technical Report Series No. 522, Energy and protein requirements, Geneva. 1973.
[17] HAJÓS, GY. and A. HALÁSZ, Acta Alimentaria **11** (1982) 189—197.
[18] BARÁTH, Á., and A. HALÁSZ, in: Amino acid composition and biological value of cereal proteins. Ed. by R. LÁSZTITY and M. HIDVÉGI, pp. 337—345. D. Reidel Publ. Co. and Akadémiai Kiadó, Budapest 1985.
[19] HIDVÉGI, M., and F. BÉKÉS, Ibid., pp. 205—286.
[20] HALÁSZ, A., Élelmezési Ipar **40** (1986) 361—367.

Prof. Dr. R. LÁSZTITY, Technical University Budapest, Department of Biochemistry and Food Technology, H-1521 Budapest, PF 91, Hungary; M. A. EL SHAFEI, M. B. ABDEL SAMEI, F. S. HATOUR, and M. LABIB, Agriculture Biochemistry Department, Faculty of Agriculture, El Minia University, El Minia, Egypt

Received May 25, 1987

Rezensionen

K.-H. Bässler, W. L. Fekl und K. Lang: **Grundbegriff der Ernährungslehre, 4. Aufl.** 211 Seiten, 20 Abb., 68 Tab. Springer-Verlag, Berlin u. a. 1988. Preis: 27,50 DM.

Das Taschenbuch, das nach dem Anliegen der Autoren lediglich ein Fundament für die Beschäftigung mit dem Fachgebiet legen möchte, behandelt Grundlagen der Verdauung und Resorption, quantitative Aspekte (Energiebilanzen), qualitative Gesichtspunkte (spezielle stoffliche Darstellungen), verschieden wirkende Nahrungsinhaltsstoffe (Schad- und Zusatzstoffe), Wechselbeziehungen zwischen Fehlernährung und Krankheiten sowie die Diätetik und besondere Ernährungsformen. Je ein kurzes Kapitel über den Hungerstoffwechsel, Postaggressionsstoffwechsel und Probleme der Welternährung sind zur schnellen Orientierung vor vertiefender Lektüre geeignet. Das Kapitel über Lipide wurde überarbeitet, wobei allerdings nicht an die neuen Rapszüchtungen gedacht wurde. Das Ballaststoffkapitel sagt dem Rezensenten ebensowenig zu wie die in Inhalt und Aussage einfach zu spärlichen Kapitel über Schad- und Zusatzstoffe und Sekundärprodukte der Verarbeitung. Die moderne Nomenklatur sollte in die nächste Auflage Eingang finden. In einer umfangmäßig so begrenzten Schrift dürfte die Auswahl der Fakten schwer gefallen sein. Die Autoren verzichten deshalb auf viele chemische Aspekte, haben aber etwas weiterführende Literatur (von der es sicher informativere und modernere Schriften gäbe, mitunter auch neuere Auflage gibt) beigefügt. R. Macholz

Evaluation of certain veterinary drug residues in food. Thirty-second Report of the Joint FAO/WHO Expert Committee on Food Additives (WHO Technical Report Series 763). 40 Seiten. World Health Organization, Geneva 1988, Preis: 6,— Swfr.

Die Expertenkommission hat sich auf ihrer Zusammenkunft im Juni 1987 mit der Definition für diese Stoffe und mit den zu ihrer Bewertung notwendigen Informationen (Anwendungsgebiet; analytische, pharmakologische Daten, Kenntnisse zum Metabolismus, zur Toxizität und zum Rückstandsverhalten unter Feldbedingungen, zum ADI u. a.) befaßt. An Einzelsubstanzen betrachteten die Experten Chloramphenicol (Ersatz in der Behandlung lebensmittelproduzierender Tiere gefordert!), Estradiol-17β, Progesteron, Testosteron, Trenbolonacetat (temporary ADI 0—0,1 µg/kg KM) und Zeranol. Mit Ausnahme für die endogenen Wachstumspromotoren werden Monographien angekündigt. Zu diesen Stoffen werden nur Rückstandsdaten veröffentlicht (FAO Food Nutr. Paper 41, FAO/WHO, Rom 1988). R. Macholz

F. Geiss: **Fundamentals of Thin Layer Chromatography (Planar Chromatography).** 482 Seiten, 202 Abb., 40 Tab. Dr. Alfred Hüthig Verlag, Heidelberg, Basel, New York 1987. Preis: 192,— DM.

Der Autor versucht mit dem vorliegenden Buch Vorurteile, die gegenüber der planaren Dünnschichtchromatographie bestanden und bestehen, auszuräumen und die umfangreichen Möglichkeiten des Einsatzes der Methode, aber auch ihre Grenzen darzustellen. Dieser Vorsatz kann als gelungen bezeichnet werden. Es ist insbesondere hervorzuheben, daß es dem Autor gelungen ist, ein ausgewogenes Verhältnis zwischen Theorie und Hinweisen für den Praktiker einzuhalten.

Das Buch gliedert sich in 12 Kapitel. In der Einleitung werden Vor- und Nachteile der Dünnschichtchromatographie im Vergleich zur Säulenchromatographie dargestellt. Die folgenden Abschnitte behandeln u. a. Lösungsmittelfluß und Schichtqualität, Sorbentien und deren Aktivität, Laufmittel, Temperatureinflüsse und weitere beeinflussende Faktoren, quantitative Dünnschichtchromatographie.

Aus der Sicht des Rezensenten ist das Buch eine Bereicherung der analytischen Literatur und selbst für den langjährigen Praktiker eine Fundgrube neuer Erkenntnisse. M. Kujawa

Die Nahrung 32 (1988) 9, 875—879

Research Institute for Food Industry, Havana, Cuba

Quality of canned grapefruit juice produced in Cuba during four seasons

J. Pino and Ana M. Cabrera

Canned single-strength grapefruit juice samples were collected biweekly from the main producing plant in Cuba during the 1980—81 to 1983—84 seasons. They were analyzed for °Brix, acid, naringin and limonin content and evaluated for sensory quality. Average values for each quality factor vary from season to season. Better sensory quality was found in samples with high Brix/acid ratio and lower bitter compounds content. No correlation relationship was found between Brix, Brix/acid ratio, naringin and limonin. The first 3 are the main quality factors related to grapefruit juice flavour.

Introduction

With increasing citrus production in Cuba the quality of processed citrus juice has become an important concern for the grower, processor and consumer. In reply, the Ministry for Food Industry has started a citrus quality improvement programme, This investigation, part of the programme, is one of several concerning grapefruit juice.

State standards regulate manufacture of grapefruit juice products in Cuba [1]. Requirements for these products include sensorial quality (out of 20 total points): 11 for flavour, 5 for appearance and 4 for odour. "Good" flavour required for Cuban grapefruit juice is defined as that typical of freshly-extracted juice from mature, well-ripened grapefruit. Other quality factors include: minimum °Brix, minimum and maximum percent acid, maximum suspended pulp and maximum recoverable oil. Regulations in Florida also include maximums for the content of the bitter compounds naringin and limonin [2] which occur naturally.

Objectives of this study were to determine the following: a) degree of variability of quality factors between various citrus seasons, b) selected chemical and physical factors for the juice, and c) possible relationships between these factors.

Material and methods

Samples were collected on a biweekly basis from the main producing plant in Cuba of canned single strength grapefruit juice during the 1980—81 to 1983—84 seasons. A total of 58, 60, 62 and 56 samples were collected and analyzed in each season. Samples were packed in 542 ml cans.

Juices were analyzed for °Brix and % citric acid in the usual manner [3, 4], naringin by HPLC [5, 6] and limonin by thin-layer chromatography procedure [7]. Sensory quality was evaluated by a selected 6 member panel using a 20 point scale (quality score) for appearance, odour and flavour, 5 points for each. By means of conversion factors of 1, 0.8 and 2.2 for each attribute, the addition of the 3 is converted in a 20 total point scale [8].

Results and discussion

Table 1 gives the average, maximum and minimum values for the quality factors of commercial, canned, single-strength grapefruit juice packed in 1980—81 to 1983—84 seasons. Maximum and minimum values show large variations in all of the values for the seasons. The average values for °Brix, % acid and their ratio vary from season to season. Bitter compounds also vary between seasons, although limonin has been determined during the last two seasons only.

Quality score is defined in terms of a ponderated average of the main attributes of the juice. As shown in Table 1 naringin and limonin values tend to be higher and quality scores were lower for the 1982—83 season, mainly due to lower odour and flavour scores. On the other hand, the Brix/acid ratio was lowest for that season. The opposite behaviour was observed in 1983—84 season. Therefore in terms of seasonal averages, high quality score juices are associated with high Brix/acid ratio and low bitter compounds content. Similar results were found by United States' researchers [9—11]. The relationship between the above quality factors is better observed in Fig. 1 based on averages for the 1982—83 and 1983—84 seasons. These results suggest that the easiest way to increase quality of grapefruit juice is to increase Brix/acid ratio from 7.8 to 8.8.

Data for the 4 seasons was analyzed statistically for correlation among the quality factors. The correlation matrix is shown in Table 2. Many significant correlations were noted but with most showed relatively low correlation coefficients. With the exception of appearance-flavour, all sensory factors correlated among them. Quality score had a positive correlation with °Brix, Brix/acid ratio and negative with naringin content. No correlation was found with limonin content for the two seasons studied. Therefore limonin is an uncertain indicator of juice quality which is contrary to the results of other researchers [9, 12] who have found

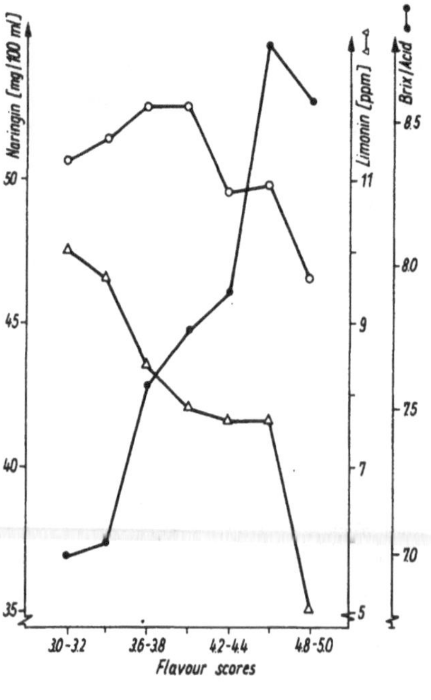

Fig. 1
Relationship between flavour, Brix/acid ratio, naringin and limonin content in commercial, canned, single-strength grapefruit juice.

Table 1
Average, maximum and minimum values for some quality analyses of commercial, canned, single-strength grapefruit juice

Quality factor	Average				Maximum				Minimum			
	80—81	81—82	82—83	83—84	80—81	81—82	82—83	83—84	80—81	81—82	82—83	83—84
°Brix (B)	9.4	9.8	9.3	10.1	11.0	11.7	9.8	11.2	8.5	9.1	8.8	9.0
% Acid (A)	1.24	1.28	1.24	1.32	1.51	1.52	1.51	1.67	1.07	0.98	0.89	1.06
Ratio B/A	7.71	7.69	7.53	7.80	10.1	10.1	10.4	9.10	6.20	6.36	6.09	6.28
Naringin [mg/100 ml]	50.7	43.6	51.3	50.4	58.9	58.9	61.4	64.6	36.0	32.3	40.8	38.5
Limonin [ppm]	—	—	8.8	7.5	—	—	15.0	15.0	—	—	2.5	2.5
Quality score	15.5	15.6	14.9	16.7	17.7	17.9	17.1	19.2	13.3	10.9	12.7	13.6
— Appearance	4.6	4.8	4.1	4.5	5.0	5.0	5.0	5.0	4.2	4.2	3.0	3.8
— Odour	3.9	3.9	3.5	4.0	4.3	4.4	4.0	4.6	3.3	3.3	2.3	3.3
— Flavour	3.5	3.5	3.1	4.1	4.2	4.5	4.0	4.8	2.7	1.6	2.3	3.3

Table 2
Correlation matrix between the quality factors of commercial, canned, single-strength grapefruit juice ($n = 236$)

Quality factor	1	2	3	4	5	6	7	8	9
1. Appearance		0.32**	0.03	0.44**	0.22**	0.04	0.08	—0.14*	—0.14
2. Odour			0.46**	0.70**	0.16*	—0.03	0.10	—0.15*	—0.12
3. Flavour				0.88**	0.16*	—0.09	0.18**	—0.10	—0.18
4. Quality score					0.23	—0.07	0.19**	—0.16*	—0.19
5. °Brix (B)						—0.38**	0.20**	—0.07	0.11
6. % Acid (A)							—0.75**	0.08	0.17
7. Ratio B/A								—0.08	—0.15
8. Naringin									0.19
9. Limonin[1]									

[1] limonin content only for 1982—83 and 1983—84 seasons ($n \doteq 118$)
* $p < 0.05$ ** $p < 0.01$

that limonin content has a more negative effect on grapefruit juice flavour than naringin. However, for a quality study on retail canned grapefruit juice, TING et al. [13] found naringin assayed by HPLC methodology, but not naringin by the traditional Davis test correlated with flavour as did limonin at the same confidence level. Results of the present study would indicate that naringin contributes more to the bitterness of Cuban grapefruit juice than limonin according to panelists.

The above results suggest that further research to lower levels of naringin in commercial grapefruit juice to diminish negative effects of this compound on juice quality would be worthwhile.

Results of naringin and limonin analyses have shown that there is no correlation between the concentrations of these bitter compounds with other quality factors, thus suggesting that the kinetics of bitter compounds accumulation are independent from each other. This lack of correlation was observed by MANSELL et al. [14] in Florida grapefruit juice.

Overall, the study suggested that reduction of bitterness with an increase in Brix/acid ratio would increase consumer acceptability.

Zusammenfassung

J. PINO und ANA M. CABRERA: Qualität von in Kuba hergestelltem eingedostem Grapefruitjuice aus 4 Ernteperioden

Eingedoste nicht-konzentrierte Grapefruitjuice-Proben wurden während der Ernteperioden von 1980/81 bis 1983/84 zweiwöchentlich beim kubanischen Hauptproduzenten entnommen. Sie wurden analysiert hinsichtlich °Brix, Säure-, Naringin- und Limoningehalt; darüber hinaus wurde die sensorische Qualität beurteilt. Die Durchschnittswerte für jeden Qualitätsfaktor variieren von Saison zu Saison. Eine bessere sensorische Qualität wurde in Proben mit hohem Brix/Säure-Verhältnis und niedrigem Gehalt an Bitterstoffen gefunden. Es waren keine korrelativen Beziehungen zwischen Brix, Brix/Säure-Verhältnis, Naringin und Limonin zu finden. Die ersten 3 Faktoren sind für die Qualität des Flavours von Grapefruitjuice am wichtigsten.

Резюме

Й. ПИНО и АНА М. КАБРЕРА: Качество изготовленного на кубе расфасованного в банки сока грейпфрутов 4 периодов уборки

Расфасованные в банки неконцентрированные пробы сока грейпфрутов в периодах урожая 1980/81 до 1983/84 гг. каждые 2 недели брали у главного продуцента на Кубе. Они анализировались в отношении °Brix, содержания кислоты, нарингина и лимонина; кроме того оценивалось сенсорное качество. Средные данные каждого качественного колеблются со сезона на сезон. Более хорошее сенсорное качество наблюдалось в пробах с высоким соотношением Brix/кислота и низким содержанием горьких веществ. Не найдены корреляционные отношения между параметрами Brix, Brix/кислота, нарингин и лиминин. Первые 3 фактора являются наиважнейшими для качества флевора сока грейпфрутов.

References

[1] Standard State Committe (CEN). Quality standard for single-strength grapefruit juice NC 77—10 Cuba (1980).
[2] State of Florida, Dep. of Citrus. Official rules affecting the Florida citrus industry (1982).
[3] Standard State Committee (CEN). Standard method for soluble solids NC 77-22-4 Cuba (1982).

[4] Standard State Committee (CEN). Standard method for titrable acid NC 77-22-7 Cuba (1982).
[5] FISHER, J., J. Agric. Food Chem. **24**, 898 (1976).
[6] PINO, J., and A. LAGUNA, Rev. Cienc. Tecnol. Alim. 2 (in press) (1987).
[7] MAIER, V., and E. GRANT, J. Agric. Food Chem. **18**, 250 (1970).
[8] MINAL. Sensory evaluation. Procedure for fruit juices. Instruction SCC 2-15 Cuba (1979).
[9] DOUGHERTY, M., and J. FISHER, Proc. Fla. State Hort. Soc. **90**, 168 (1977).
[10] ROUSEFF, R., S. BARROS, M. DOUGHERTY and S. MARTIN, Proc. Fla. State Hort. Soc. **93**, 286 (1980).
[11] FELLERS, P., G. DEJAGER, M. POOLE, E. HILL and P. MITTAL, J. Food Sci. **51**, 417 (1986).
[12] BARROS, S., J. DAVIS, M. DOUGHERTY and J. GRIFFITHS, Proc. Fla. State Hort. Soc. **96**, 316 (1983).
[13] TING, S., and J. MCALLISTER, Proc. Fla. State Hort. Soc. **90**, 170 (1977).
[14] MANSELL, R., C. MCINTOSH and J. VEST, J. Agric. Food Chem. **31**, 156 (1983).

Dr. J. A. PINO, Research Institute for Food Industry (IIIA), Ave. Rancho Boyeros Km $3^1/_2$, Cerro, Havana, Cuba

Received June 3, 1987

Rezensionen

W. FRIEDRICH: **Handbuch der Vitamine.** 657 Seiten, 168 Abb. und Formelschemata, 227 Tab. Urban & Schwarzenberg, München, Wien, Baltimore 1987. Preis: 298,— DM.

Das hervorragend ausgestattete Werk ist nicht nur die überzeugende Dokumentation einer Renaissance der Vitaminforschung. Es nötigt auch höchsten Respekt ab angesichts der gewaltigen enzyklopädischen Arbeitsleistung, die sich ein einzelner zugemutet und mit einiger Bravour im Wettlauf mit der Zeit bewältigt hat. 4420 Literaturstellen hat der Autor aufbereitet und dabei nur zu einem geringen Teil noch auf Publikationen aus den 70er Jahren zurückgegriffen. Nachgetragen hat er am Ende weitere 370 Literaturhinweise für die Jahre 1984 bis 1986 und dies mit voller Titelangabe.

Vorangestellt ist ein Einführungskapitel mit weitgehend tabellarischer Struktur. In ihm werden in vergleichender Betrachtung und leicht überschaubar bereits die wichtigsten Informationen vermittelt. Es folgen dann spezielle Kapitel über die einzelnen, heute nomenklaturgemäß als Vitamine angesehenen 13 Nährstoffe. Nach einem gleichbleibenden, wenn auch nicht immer konsequent durchgehaltenen Algorithmus mit breit gefächerter Gliederung werden die chemischen, physikalischen, biochemischen und physiologischen Grundlagen abgehandelt und aus klinischer Sicht angeborene Stoffwechselstörungen sowie pharmakologische, therapeutische und toxische Wirkungen aufgezeigt. Mensch und Tier werden gleichermaßen in die Betrachtung einbezogen. Jedem Kapitel angefügt ist eine alphabetisch nach Autorennamen geordnete Bibliographie.

Der Handbuchcharakter und das verfolgte Ziel, den gegenwärtigen Wissensstand vollständig zu erfassen und wiederzugeben, bringen es wohl mit sich, daß es vielfach zu Redundanz, Überschneidungen und selbst zu Widersprüchen kommt. Es ist nicht ganz leicht und nach Lage der Dinge auch nicht in allen Belangen möglich, aus der Fülle mitgeteilter Daten und Befunde verbindliche Lehrmeinungen abzuleiten. Zu sehr ist die Vitaminforschung wieder in Fluß geraten, und es ist schon erstaunlich, welche Kenntnislücken sich beim Studium jüngster Ergebnisse noch immer auftun.

Auf Verbindungen, die unter besonderen Umständen Vitamincharakter annehmen können oder solche, die zwar nicht bzw. nicht mehr zu den Vitaminen gerechnet, die aber in der Laienpresse gelegentlich hochgespielt werden und die auch forschungsseitig durchaus nicht abgetan sind, geht der Autor nicht ein. Man mag das bedauern, weil man der Auseinandersetzung deshalb nicht enthoben ist, doch man muß es in Anbetracht wichtigerer Bestandsaufnahmen akzeptieren. Was der Rezensent mehr bedauert, ist die selbst auferlegte Beschränkung hinsichtlich des Sachregisters. Der Verweis auf sehr ausführliche Inhaltsverzeichnisse zu den einzelnen Kapiteln ist weder hinreichend nützlich noch tröstlich. B. GASSMANN

T. LINDL und J. BAUER: **Zell- und Gewebekultur.** Einführung in die Grundlagen sowie ausgewählte Methoden und Anwendungen. 191 Seiten, 41 Abb., 29 Tab. Gustav Fischer Verlag, Stuttgart, New York 1987. Preis: 36,— DM.

In 14 Kapiteln wird dem Leser eine Übersicht über die hauptsächlichsten Belange der Zell- und Gewebekultur vermittelt. Zunächst werden die prinzipiellen Anforderungen an Zellkulturlaboratorien, Grundsätze der sterilen Labortechnik sowie Grundlagen der Zell- und Gewebekulturtechnik vermittelt. Im Anschluß daran werden spezielle Zelltypen, wie Invertebraten- und Pflanzenzellen, an verschiedenen Beispielen behandelt. Spezielle Methodiken und Anwendungsgebiete schließen den fachlichen Teil ab. Hier sind vor allem die Anwendungen in der Toxikologie, Gentechnik und Virusherstellung zu nennen und Methodiken der Klonierung und Wachstums-Synchronisation hervorzuheben. Die letzten zwei Kapitel bilden ein knappes Lexikon der wichtigsten Fachtermini und eine Aufstellung von Bezugsquellen und Lieferfirmen von Chemikalien, Materialien und Geräten. Die einzelnen Kapitel sind in der Art aufgebaut, daß vom theoretischen Hintergrund zu laborpraktischen Einzelheiten übergegangen wird, welche eindeutig den Schwerpunkt des Buches bilden. Eine rasche Orientierung wird durch graphische Hervorhebung von Laborrezepturen erleichtert, die durch umfangreiches Tabellenmaterial ergänzt werden. Jedem Kapitel ist ein Verzeichnis der wichtigsten weiterführenden Literatur nachgestellt. Inhaltlich stehen tierische Zell- und Gewebekulturen im Vordergrund. Nur in einem Kapitel werden pflanzliche Systeme behandelt. Hier kommt es leider — im Gegensatz zu den übrigen Darstellungen — in Folge hoher Abstraktion zu manchen Unklarheiten (Besonderheiten der Pflanzenzelle in vitro, Einfluß von Licht, Einsatz von Phytohormonen). Dennoch vermittelt das Buch Studenten, Laboranten und „Einsteigern" ein schnelles Zurechtfinden auf diesem Gebiet und behält als Nachschlagewerk in der Laborpraxis seinen Wert. H. HERMERSDÖRFER

Die Nahrung 32 (1988) 9, 881—888

Food Science and Technology Department,
Faculty of Agriculture, Alexandria University,
Alexandria, Egypt

Preparation, foaming, electrophoretic patterns and storage of concentrated liquid eggs

A. A. DAMIR, ESMAT M. EL-ZALAKI and T. M. IBRAHIM

A new egg product was recommended for bakery goods requiring high foaming capacity and stability such as sponge cake. Aerating of eggs was stabilised by sugaring at a rate of one part of sugar to two parts of eggs, followed by pasteurization and evaporation to yield a concentrated product of 69—70% total soluble solids. Two new bands appeared in the electrophoretic pattern of eggs after pasteurization and evaporation, which could be used as an evaluation for heat treatment of eggs. The concentrated liquid eggs maintained their foaming properties upon storage for a long period at room temperature. The free fatty acids, peroxide value and thiobarbaturic acid value started to increase in the product after three months of storage. Microbiological examination indicated that it was free of *Salmonellae*.

Introduction

Eggs are one of the few foods which are used throughout the world; thus the egg industry is an important segment of food manufacture. There are basically three types of egg products, namely, dried, frozen and liquid [14]. ROLFES [24] found that the whole egg powder was not stable even when the moisture content was as low as 2%, when objectionable off-flavour and colour changes developed. Moreover, damage caused by the drying process affected the aeration function and deterioration occurred on storage. FEENEY et al. [4] observed that frozen egg products underwent changes in yolk consituents during freezing and thawing which affected their function properties.

Certain processing and storage conditions should be considered to preserve the quality of the frozen products [6]. Liquid egg products are processed for immediate consumption, drying and freezing or for tank shipment [9]. ZABIC et al. [27] found that cakes prepared by using freeze-dried whole eggs exhibited undesirable texture and tendernes qualities and received slightly lower scores for flavour. EGAN et al. [6] reported that sugar was the most effective ingredient in protecting the foaming capacity of egg due to stabilization of the lipoprotein.

In this work, an attempt was carried out to prepare a concentrated liquid eggs product containing sugar, for bakery products and to demonstrate physical, chemical and microbiological changes that occur during storage.

Materials and methods

Fresh eggs of Leghorn L.H. hens collected from the farm of the Faculty of Agriculture, University of Alexandria, were used.

Preparation of concentrated liquid eggs

The clean fresh eggs were broken and the contents were gently blended with a wire whip. Refined cane sugar powder was added gradually by stirring in a proportion of one part by weight of sugar to two parts of eggs. Pasteurization was carried out at 60 °C for 3 min [19]. For concentration the mixture was allowed to evaporate with continuous stirring at 60 °C to yield a product of 69—70% total soluble solids as determined refractometrically. The concentrated product was kept in glass containers and stored at room temperature for further study.

Foaming properties

The foaming capacity and foam stability of homogenized whole eggs were measured according to [17], with some modifications. A 20 g sample was blended by an electric blender (Mkzolon, Matsushita Electric Trading Co., LTD, Japan) at medium speed for 3 min. The mixture was poured into 100 ml graduate measuring cylinder and the total volume measured after 30 s was considered as foam capacity. The foam stability was determined 15, 30, 60 and 120 min after pouring into the cylinder. The effect of the addition of 10, 20, 30, 40, 50, 60 and 70% of sugar on the foam capacity and stability of eggs was also determined.

In the case of the concentrated liquid eggs containing 50% sugar, the product was diluted so as to simulate the fresh mixture. 30 g of the resulting mixture (20 g of eggs and 10 g of sugar) were used to determine the foam capacity and stability.

Chemical examination

The free fatty acids of concentrated liquid eggs fat were determined as percentage of oleic acid according to [1]. The peroxide value was determined according to the method described by [22]. Thiobarbituric acid value was calculated as mg malonaldehyde per kg of sample according to [16].

Microbiological examination

Serial dilutions of a representative sample of concentrated liquid eggs were made and sterilized nutrient agar (Difco) was used as culture medium for total bacterial count [21]. Detection of *Salmonellae* was carried out as described by [21].

Polyacrylamide gel electrophoresis

A volume of 50 ml each of homogenized fresh, pasteurized and concentrated liquid eggs was stirred with cold acetone (1:5, V/V) for 1 h, centrifuged, and the precipitate treated twice with cold acetone. 250 mg of the acetone dried material were shaken for 1 h with 5 ml of distilled water in a screw cap test tube, then centrifuged. The supernatant was stained with few drops of Amido black 10B. Gel of 6% acrylamide and N,N methylene bis-acrylamide and electrophoresis buffer of tris-borate (pH 8.9) were prepared as described by [26]. Electrophoresis was performed in PANTA-PHOR apparatus using 3 mm slab gel. The gel was removed and stained with coomassie Brilliant blue R250 and destained by acetic acid:methanol:water (1:6:14, V:V:V) overnight.

Results and discussions

The effects of various concentrations of sugar on foaming capacity and foam stability of whole liquid eggs was improved by sugar addition. This may be due to the stabilization by egg lipoproteins according to [7]. Maximum increase in foam capacity was noted at sugar concentration of 50% whereas at 60 and 70% slight increase in volume was obtained as compared with the results in the absence of added sugar. The slight increase in volume at 60 and 70% sugar was most likely due to the increase in viscosity of the resulting foam. The foam stability after 15 and 30 min in the presence or absence of sugar was generally higher than that after 60 or 120 min. The addition of sugar at a concentration of 10% improved the foaming stability of whole liquid eggs. The foam stability was almost similar at sugar concentration of 20 and 30% then it slightly increased at 40%, reaching a maximum at 50%, after which it decreased as the sugar concentration increased to 60 and 70% (Table 1).

In most foams, the liquid phase existed as lamellae between adjacent bubbles. Instability of foam was indicated by drainage of liquid from the lamellae, and by the rupture of bubbles. This was found to be dependent on surface viscosity, capillary forces, film thickness and orientation of surface active solutes such as carbohydrates and proteins according to [23]. This could explain the adverse effects of sugar at high levels of 60 and 70% on foam capacity and stability of whole liquid eggs. Therefore, at higher levels of added sugar, it was evident that the whipping time should be increased.

The foam capacity and stability of egg containing 50, 60 and 70% sugar were increased by prolonging the whipping time (Table 2). The same foam capacity was nearly obtained after 5 and 7 min of whipping at the three sugar levels. However, the resulting foams after 7 min appeared to be more stable especially at 70% sugar concentration. Generally the 50% sugar concentration had higher improving effect on the foaming capacity as compared with the 60 and 70% sugar levels.

In sponge cake formulation, the proportion of sugar used was about 70% of the egg weight [4]. Thus, it was recommended that sugar was first added to egg at a concentration of 50% and whipping was carried out for 5 min in order to obtain the highest foaming capacity, followed by the addition of 20% sugar where whipping was continued for further 2 min. This procedure gave both high foaming capacity and stability.

Fig. 1 shows the electrophoretic patterns of fresh, pasteurized and evaporated whole egg containing 50% sugar. Three bands were demonstrated in fresh egg prior to pasteurization. When egg was heated to 60 °C for pasteurization, two new protein bands appeared, which may be due to the dissociation of macroglobulin protein [5], and/or to the interaction between macroglobulin and lysozyme [20]. The pattern of the protein bands in the concentrated

Table 1
Effect of sugar concentration on the foaming capacity and foam stability of whole liquid eggs

Sugar concentration [%]	Foam capacity [ml] after 30 s	Increase [%]	Foam stability after			
			15 min	30 min	60 min	120 min
0	60	300	59	57	56	54
10	70	350	68	66	61	59
20	71	355	70	70	67	61
30	72	360	71	70	68	61
40	75	375	74	73	70	65
50	78	390	78	77	76	72
60	66	330	66	66	64	64
70	66	330	66	66	65	64

Table 2
Effect of whipping time and sugar concentration on foam capacity and foam stability of whole liquid eggs

Sugar conc. [%]	Whipping time [min]														
	3	5	7	3				5				7			
	Foam capacity [ml] after 30 s			Foam stability [ml] after				Foam stability [ml] after				Foam stability [ml] after			
				15 min	30 min	60 min	120 min	15 min	30 min	60 min	120 min	15 min	30 min	60 min	120 min
50	78	90	90	78	77	76	71	90	88	85	77	90	90	86	81
60	66	84	84	66	66	63	62	83	82	80	77	84	83	83	81
70	66	85	85	66	66	65	62	85	85	82	80	85	85	85	84

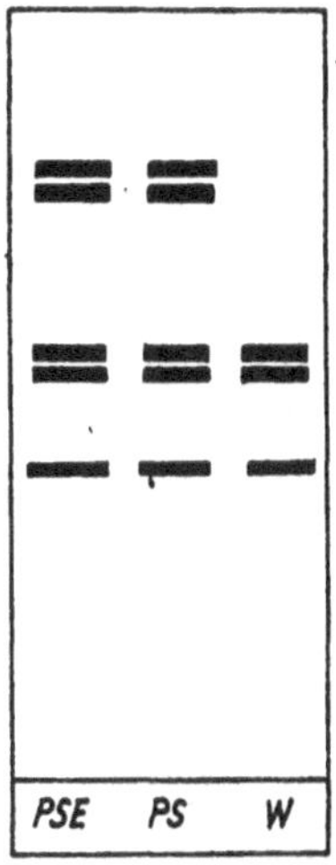

Fig. 1
Electrophoretic patterns of liquid whole eggs (w), pasteurized sugared whole eggs (PS), and pasteurized evaporated concentrated liquid eggs (PSE)

egg product was almost the same as that of pasteurized egg. However, the intensity of the new protein bands was reduced on further heat treatment during evaporation. Heat sensitivity of egg proteins during evaporation, resulting in partial denaturation, could be responsible for the reduction of the band intensity. SATO et al. [25] and NAKAMURA et al. [19] showed that the intensities of macaroglobulin protein bands in electrophoretic pattern of egg white were decreased on heating at 60 °C for long periods.

Accordingly, one may use this new band formation as an indicator for heat treatment of liquid whole egg.

Changes in concentrated eggs during storage

The foam capacity of eggs slightly decreased during the preparation of the concentrate (Table 3). This may be due to the heat treatment used during concentrated eggs process.

Table 3
Changes in foam capacity and foam stability of concentrated eggs containing 50% sugar during preparation and storage at room temperature

Storage time [month]	Foam capacity [ml] after 30 s	Foam stability [ml] after			
		15 min	30 min	60 min	120 min
Before pasteurization and evaporation	78	78	77	76	71
After pasteurization and evaporation	75	75	75	73	70
1	75	75	74	72	70
2	74	74	74	70	68
3	75	75	74	71	67
4	74	74	74	70	67
5	70	70	70	65	62
6	68	68	67	62	60

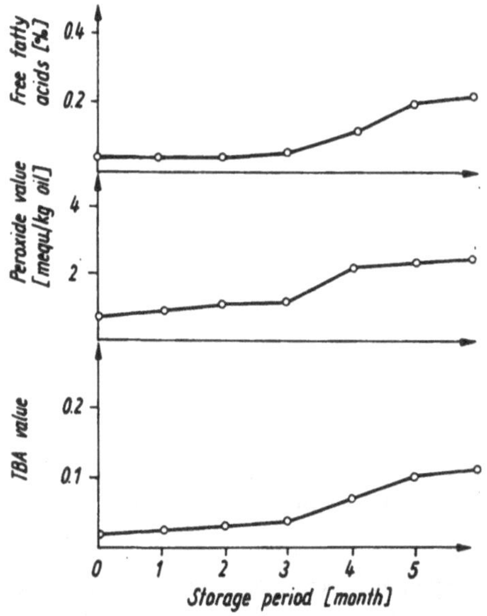

Fig. 2
Changes in free fatty acids, peroxide value and thiobarbituric acid value in concentrated eggs during storage at room temperature

Garibaldi et al. [8] found that an ovomucin-lysozyme complex formation during heating was related to loss of foaming properties of egg. Baldwin [2] reported that the mild heat treatment used in egg pasteurization caused the whipping time to increase and also decreased both foam volume and stability.

No considerable changes in both foam capacity and stability of concentrated eggs were observed during storage at room temperature for 4 months, after which a slight decrease was obtained upon storage for 6 months. The protective effect of the added sugar on the foaming capacity of eggs was mainly due to their reaction to the protein and phospholipid leading to the stabilization of the lipoproteins according to [15].

The foaming capacity of shell eggs remained unchanged after storage for 10 and 20 days at 25 °C and 4 °C respectively [12]. While that of dehydrated or freeze-dried eggs was considerably lowered [24, 10]. Concentrated eggs maintained their foaming properties after preparation and even upon storage for a long period, reflecting the advantage of concentrated liquid eggs as compared with the other means of egg preservation.

The free fatty acids of concentrated eggs rose slightly through the first 3 months of storage, followed by sharp increase (Fig. 2). Prolonging storage time resulted in obvious increase in the peroxide value particularly after 3 months of storage.

The thiobarbituric acid value (TBA) of concentrated eggs was gradually increased during storage at room temperature. Though the increase of the peroxide value was not detected markedly except after 3 months of storage, yet the TBA value started to increase from the first month of storage. The results agree with those reported by [15]. Concentrated liquid eggs gave a bacterial count of 90×10^3/g.

ICMSF [13] recommended that pasteurized whole egg should have a general viable count of less than 10^6/g, and that *Salmonellae* should be absent from 125 g. Although the total microbial count increased gradually through the storage period, it did not exceed that recommended by [13]. No *Salmonellae* was detected in the concentrated liquid eggs either before pasteurization or after pasteurization and storage for 6 months.

In conclusion, the aeration of eggs can be stabilized by at a rate of one part of sugar to two parts of eggs, followed by pasteurization and evaporation to yield concentrated liquid eggs suitable for baking products requiring high foaming properties such as sponge cake. In addition, such products facilitate processing, are time saving and are more sanitary with the added advantage of being able to be stored at room temperature for long periods without considerable deterioration.

Zusammenfassung

A. A. DAMIR, ESMAT M. EL-ZALAKI und T. M. IBRAHIM: Herstellung, Verschäumung, elektrophoretisches Verhalten und Lagerung von konzentriertem Flüssigei

Für Backwaren, die eine hohe Schaumkapazität und -stabilität erfordern, wird ein neues Eiprodukt empfohlen. Die Verschäumung von Eiern wird durch Zusatz von 1 Teil Zucker zu 2 Teilen Ei stabilisiert mit anschließender Pasteurisierung und Einengen zu einem Produkt mit 69—70% Trockenmasse. Durch diesen Prozeß treten im Elektropherogramm zwei neue Banden auf, die als Nachweis einer Wärmebehandlung von Eiern herangezogen werden können. Das flüssige Eikonzentrat behält seine Verschäumungseigenschaften während einer langen Lagerungszeit bei Raumtemperatur. Nach 3monatiger Lagerung beginnen der Gehalt an freien Fettsäuren, die Peroxidzahl und die Thiobarbitursäurezahl im Produkt zuzunehmen. Mikrobiologische Untersuchungen zeigen, daß Salmonellen nicht nachweisbar sind.

Резюме

А. А. Дамир, Эсмат М. Эль-Залаки и Т. М. Ибрахим: Получение, вспенивание, электрофоретическое поведение и хранение концентрированного жидкого яйца

Для кондитерских изделий, требующих высокой емкости и прочности пены предлагается новый яичмый продукт. Вспенивание яиц стабилизируется добавлением I части сахара к 2 частям яиц с последующей пастеризации и концентрировании до продукта со содержанием сухой массой 69—70%. В результате этого процесса в электроферограмме появляются две новые полосы, которые являются доказательством тепловой обработки яиц. Жидкий яичный концентрат сохраняет вспенивающие свойства во время длительного хранения при комнатной температуре. После трехмесячного хранения содержание свободный жирных кислот, перекисное число и число тиобарбитуровой кислоты в продукте повышаются.

References

[1] Official Methods of Analysis, A.O.A.C., Association of Official Analytical Chemists, Washington, D.C., U.S.A., 1980.
[2] BALDWIN, R. E., in: Egg Science and Technology. Ed. by W. S. STADELMAN and O. J. COTTERILL, AVI, Pub. Co., Inc., Westport, Conn., 1977.
[3] BERGQUIST, D. H., in: Egg Science and Technology. Ed. by W. S. STADELMAN and O. J. COTTERILL, AVI, Pub. Co., Inc., Westport, Conn., 1977.
[4] DAMIR, A. A., K. EL-SAYED and N. M. EL-SHIMI, Zagazic J. Agric. Res. Bull., 415 (1981).
[5] DONOVAN, J. W., C. J. MAPES, J. G. DAVIS and R. D. HAMBURG, Biochemistry **8**, 4190 (1969).
[6] EGAN, H., R. S. KIRK and R. SAWYER, Pearson's Chemical Analysis of Foods, Churchill Living-stone, Edinburgh, London 1981.
[7] FEENEY, R. E., and R. M. HILL, Advances in Food Research. Ed. by C. O. CHICHESTER, E. M. MARAK and G. F. STEWART, Academic press, New York 1960.

[8] GARIBALDI, J. A., J. W. DONOVAN, J. G. DAVIS and H. L. CIMINO, J. Food Sci. **33**, 514 (1968).
[9] GÖRNER, F., and M. VALOVICOVE, Hydinarsky Priemysel **24**, 472 (1982).
[10] HABASHY, N. H., Freeze drying of Eggs. M.Sc. Thesis, Cairo University, Cairo, Egypt, 1981.
[11] HAMZA, M. A., Electrophoretic studies on seed proteins of some Egyptian and German legumes. PH.D. Thesis, Alexandria University, Alexandria, Egypt.
[12] IBRAHEM, T. M., Use of liquid egg concentrates in sponge cakes formulation. M.Sc. Thesis, Alexandria University, Alexandria, Egypt.
[13] International Commission on Microbiological Specifications for Foods, ICMSF., International Association of Microbiological Societies, Toranto University, U.S.A., 1974.
[14] KAMAT, V. B., G. A. LAWRENCE, C. J. HART and R. YOELL, J. Sci. Food Agric. **24**, 77 (1973).
[15] KLINE, L., T. F. SUGIHARA and J. J. MEEHAN, J. Food Sci. **29**, 693 (1964).
[16] KWOV, T. W., and M. J. NORGAR, J. Food Sci. **31**, 223 (1966).
[17] LEWHON, J. T., and C. M. CATER, J. Food Sci. **36**, 372 (1971).
[18] MCCREADY, S. T., M. E. NORRIS, M. SEBRING and O. J. COTTERILL, Poultry Sci. **50**, 1810 (1971).
[19] NAKAMURA, R., O. UMEMURA and H. TAKEMOTO, Agric. biol. Chem. **43**, 325 (1979).
[20] NAKAMURA, R., and T. MATSUDA, J. Food Sci. **48**, 87 (1983).
[21] NICKERSON, J. T., and A. J. SINKEY, Microbiology of Foods and Food Processing. Amer. Elsevier Pub. Co., New York 1974.
[22] PEARSON, D., The Chemical analysis of food. Churchill Livingstone, Edinburgh, London 1976.
[23] RICHERT, S. H., J. agric. Food Chem. **27**, 665 (1979).
[24] ROLFES, T., P. CLEMENTS and A. R. WINTER, Food Technol. **9**, 569 (1955).
[25] SATO, Y., and R. NAKAMURA, Agric. biol. Chem. **41**, 2163 (1977).
[26] STEGEMANN, H., W. BÜRGERMEISTER, H. FRANKSEN and E. KROGERRECKLENFORT, Inst. für Biochemie, Messeweg 11—12, D-3300 Braunschweig, 1986.
[27] ZABIK, M. E., C. M. ANDERSON, E. M. DAVEY and N. J. WOLFE, Food Technol. **23**, 85 (1969).

Dr. A. A. DAMIR, ESMAT M. EL-ZALAKI and T. M. IBRAHIM, Food Science and Technology Department, Faculty of Agriculture, Alexandria University, Alexandria, Egypt

Received June 5, 1987

Die Nahrung 32 (1988) 9, 889—910

Zentralinstitut für Ernährung in Potsdam-Rehbrücke (Direktor: Prof. Dr. H. SCHMANDKE),
Akademie der Wissenschaften der DDR

Übersichtsartikel

Über den Einsatz von Zusatzstoffen und Stoffgemischen (Compounds) in Fleischerzeugnissen

H. PETERS, J. KROLL und B. GASSMANN

Aus ökonomischer und perspektivischer Sicht ist der Einsatz von Zusatzstoffgemischen (Compounds) und Streckstoffen in Fleischerzeugnissen eine zwangsläufige und alle Länder betreffende Entwicklung. Der vorliegende Bericht gibt eine Übersicht über Zusatzstoffe bzw. Stoffgemische, die Wurstwaren und anderen Erzeugnissen aus zerkleinertem Fleisch mit dem Ziel der Beeinflussung von Wasserbindung und Fettemulgierung zugesetzt werden. Im Hinblick darauf wird die seit 1960 erschienene Patentliteratur ausgewertet.

Über Gründe, Grundlagen und Grenzen der Streckung und Substitution von Fleisch in Wurstwaren und anderen Erzeugnissen aus zerkleinertem Fleisch ist von uns bereits früher berichtet worden [1]. Ergänzend dazu und darüber hinaus, beschäftigt sich der vorliegende Literaturbericht mit solchen Zusatzstoffen bzw. Stoffgemischen, die in den genannten Lebensmitteln einen Einfluß auf die Wasserbindung und Fettemulgierung ausüben sollen.

Es ist eine Vielzahl von Stoffen (Aromastoffe, Farbstoffe, Vitamine, Fremdproteine, Aminosäuren, Konservierungsmittel, Antioxydantien, Synergisten, Emulgatoren, Dickungsmittel, Stabilisatoren, Enzyme u. a.) bekannt, die Fleisch bzw. Fleischprodukten zugesetzt werden. Die Gründe dafür sind unterschiedlich:

- Senkung der Kosten,
- Erhöhung der Produktausbeute,
- Verbesserung der sensorischen und/oder der ernährungsphysiologischen Eigenschaften,
- Einflußnahme auf die funktionellen und technologischen Eigenschaften des Fleischbräts (z. B. Verbesserung der Wasserbindung und der Schnittfähigkeit).

In der DDR ist für die Brühwurstproduktion laut TGL 29981 prinzipiell der Einsatz von Magermilchpulver, enzymgefälltem Casein, Stärke, Gewürzen, Vollei, Volleipulver, Eiklarpulver, Polyphosphat, Ascorbinsäure sowie Koch- und Pökelsalz zulässig. Ähnliche Zusatzstoffe sind auch in anderen Industriestaaten gebräuchlich. Im folgenden wird nicht auf Salze, Pökelsalze, Pökelhilfsstoffe (z. B. Ascorbinsäure, Glucono-δ-lacton, Stärkesirup) und Kutterhilfsmittel (z. P. Phosphate, Citrate, Lactate, Tartrate) eingegangen. Die vielmehr betrachteten Zusatzstoffe dienen zur Streckung (Extender) oder Verbesserung der Bindungs- und Struktureigenschaften (Binder) von Fleischprodukten. Sie werden auch als Austauschstoffe (Substitute), Füllstoffe (Filler), Emulgatoren (Emulsifier) oder Stabilisatoren (Stabilizer) bezeichnet.

Fleisch- und Wursterzeugnisse

In Europa sind mehr als 2000 Sorten von Fleisch- und Wursterzeugnissen bekannt; zwischen 9 und 33% (im Durchschnitt 25%) des erschlachteten Fleisches werden zu verschiedenen Produkten weiterverarbeitet [2]. Dabei sind alle Erzeugnisse erfaßt, deren Herstellung mehr erfordert, als nur das Abtrennen von Tierkörper und das Zerlegen in Teilstücke. Die Palette der Fleisch- und Wursterzeugnisse ist sehr vielfältig. Dazu zählen u. a. Roh-, Brüh- und Kochwürste, Pökelwaren, Garfleischwaren, Feinkostwaren, Halb-, Dreiviertel- und Vollkonserven sowie Speckwaren. Allein im deutschsprachigen Raum kann der Verbraucher zwischen mehr als 600 Produkten wählen. Ausgangsstoff ist Fleisch verschiedener Tierarten (Schwein, Rind, Kalb, Pferd, Hammel, Geflügel u. a.) sowie unterschiedlicher anatomischer Lokalisation und chemischer Zusammensetzung. Die Produkte werden nach verschiedenen Gesichtspunkten systematisiert; eine Möglichkeit der Einteilung nach dem Grad der Zerkleinerung gibt Tab. 1 wieder.

Mit zunehmendem Zerkleinerungsgrad (Tab. 1) ergeben sich folgende Vor- und Nachteile:
— sinkende Kosten für die eingesetzten Rohstoffe,
— größere Freiheit bei der Wahl der Rohstoffe und Technologien,
— kompliziertere Mechanismen der Stabilisierung,
— relative Verringerung des Anteils an myofibrillärem Protein,
— Zunahme des Anteils von freiem (feinzerkleinertem) Fett,
— Zunahme der Möglichkeiten für den Einsatz von Zusatzstoffen [3].

Wechselwirkungen zwischen Fleischproteinen und Zusatzstoffen

Untersuchungen, die sich mit der Wirkung von Zusatzstoffen bzw. Substituten verschiedener chemischer und physikalischer Charakteristik in Fleisch- bzw. Fleischerzeugnissen beschäftigen, führen häufig zu differierenden Ergebnissen und Schlußfolgerungen. Neben Schwankungen in der Qualität und den Eigenschaften der Zusatzstoffe dürfte eine Ursache dafür die Verwendung unterschiedlicher Fleischmodellsysteme sein; diese unterscheiden sich mehr oder weniger von den praxisüblichen Verarbeitungsprozessen. Viel Zeit ist darauf verwendet worden, Labormodellsysteme zu entwickeln, die geeignet sind, vergleichbare

Tabelle 1
Einteilung von Fleisch- und Wursterzeugnissen nach dem Zerkleinerungsgrad [3]

Grad der Zerkleinerung	Beispiele
unzerkleinert (zerlegt)	Kochschinken, Keule, Lende, Zunge, Leber
grob (Wolfen, Hacken, Schneiden)	Hamburger, Corned Beef, Bratwurst, Salami, Zervelatwurst
fein (Kolloidmühle oder Schneidmischer)	Frankfurter, Wiener, Bockwurst, Lyoner, Mortadella, Leberwurst

Tabelle 2
Methoden zur Charakterisierung von Substituten bzw. Zusatzstoffen für Fleisch- und Fleischerzeugnisse

Untersuchter Bereich	Untersuchungsmethoden (Beispiele)
Zusatzstoffe in Fleischmodellsystemen	— Bestimmung der Ausbeute bzw. des Koch-, Abtropf- oder Saftverlustes — Differenzierung des Kochverlustes nach Fett-, Protein- und Wasserverlust — sensorische Prüfung — elektronenoptische Untersuchung — rheologische Untersuchung
Zusatzstoffe in vereinfachten Modellsystemen (zumeist Zweikomponentensystemen)	— Untersuchung von Löslichkeit und Quellvermögen — Untersuchung von Gelbildungsvermögen und -festigkeit — Untersuchung von Emulgierkapazität, -aktivität und -stabilität
Zusatzstoffe und deren Wechselwirkungen mit Fleischproteinen im molekularen Bereich	— SDS-Polyacrylamid-Elektrophorese — Löslichkeits- und Trübungsuntersuchungen — Chromatographische Untersuchungen — Isotopenmarkierung

Tabelle 3
Forderungen für den Einsatz funktioneller proteinreicher Zusatzstoffe in der Fleischindustrie [3]

a) allgemein

— bakteriologisch und toxikologisch unbedenklich
— milder Geruch und Geschmack
— leicht handhabbar
— neutrale pH-Reaktion
— analytisch bestimmbar
— preiswert
— salztolerant

b) funktionell

in unzerkleinertem Fleisch:	— keine Störung der Gelbildung aus Fleischproteinen — Verfestigung bei Wärmebehandlung (Gelbildung, Koagulation) — adhäsive Eigenschaften — vollständig und leicht in konzentrierten Pökellaken löslich — nicht schäumend
in grob zerkleinertem Fleisch:	— quellbar oder löslich — Verfestigung bei Wärmebehandlung (Gelbildung, Koagulation) — keine Störung der Krustenbildung
in fein zerkleinertem Fleisch:	— vollständig und leicht löslich — große Affinität zu Fett-Wasser-Grenzflächen — Bildung starker wärmestabiler Hüllen — keine Störung der Gelbildung aus Fleischproteinen

Tabelle 4
Prüfung von Zusatzstoffen in zerkleinerten Fleischerzeugnissen unter besonderer Berücksichtigung von Stoffgemischen

Nr.	Autor Patent	Zusatzstoff bzw. -stoffgemisch	Einsatz (Menge und Produkt)	Bemerkung
1	W. J. Zick US-PS 2 938 796 31. Mai 1960 B. Heller & Company	getrocknetes und entöltes *Mehl aus der Schale von Zitrusfrüchten* (Zitronen, Limonen, Orangen, Grapefruit, Tangerine) Zusammensetzung von Zitronenschalenmehl: Asche 3 ... 4% Hemicellulose 30 ... 35% Protopektin (unlösliches Pektin) 18 ... 22% andere Stoffe 8% Wasser Rest	Zitrusschalenmehl — 1% zu Frankfurtern und Bolognern — 3—4% übliche Empfehlung — 15—20% max. ohne sensorische Beeinträchtigung des Produktes	— getrocknetes und entöltes Zitrusschalenmehl zeigt gute Wasserabsorptionseigenschaften; diese sind auch bei hohen Temperaturen und während der Lagerung beständig — wirkt schon bei geringen Einsatzmengen
2	E. H. Freund und E. N. Danes US-PS 2 957 770 25. Okt. 1960 National Dairy Products Corporation	*Casein-Calcium-Phosphat-Gel:* Gel, gebildet aus der wäßrigen Lösung von 4 Komponenten: 1) Casein (handelsüblich, u. U. α-Casein) 2) Calcium-Quelle (Calcium-Caseinat, lösl. Calciumsalze, Kalk) 3) Pyrophosphat (Tetra-alkalipyrophosphat, $Na_4P_2O_7$, u. stärker saure Salze der Pyrophosphorsäure) 4) Orthophosphat (Orthophosphorsäure u. ihre Alkali- u. Calciumsalze, soweit wasserlöslich)	— Wurstprodukte, z. B. Frankfurter — nahezu optimale Gelstärke bei folgenden Anteilen: Calcium = 2× (g Casein) Pyrophosphat = 0,5× (mmol Calcium) Orthophosphat = 0,33× (mmol Calcium) — dabei ist der Anteil z. B. von Orthophosphat im Fleisch zu berücksichtigen	— α-Casein bildet (β-Casein bildet keine) Gele mit entsprechenden Mengen Calcium, Pyro- u. Orthophosphat — pH muß für Gelbildung optimal eingestellt werden (pH = 6,5 ... 7,5) — andere Polyphosphate, z. B. Hexametaphosphat, Tripolyphosphat usw. bilden keine starken Gele — Gelstärke durch die Reihenfolge der Substanzzugabe beeinflußt a) hohe Gelstärke, bei Pyrophosphatzugabe zur Casinlsg. vor der Calciumzugabe b) geringe Gelstärke: Calcium- und Orthophosphatzugabe zur

				Caseinlsg. vor Pyrophosphatzugabe — bei Mischung der Trockensubstanzen wird die Gelstärke relativ gering (evtl. Umhüllen der Calciumkomponente) — höhere Temp. liefern niedrige Gelstärken — Textur der Würste verbessert
3	L. SAIR US-PS 2 964 409 13. Dez. 1960 Griffith Laboratories	*Calciumcaseinat*	— Wurstprodukte, z. B. Frankfurter — Einsatzmenge Ca-Caseinat: 0,5 Teile auf 100 Teile Fleisch oder vorzugsweise 1 ... 8 Teile auf 100 Teile Fleisch — Gemisch von Ca- u. Na-Caseinaten	— Ca-Caseinat zeigt bessere Eigenschaften als Na-Caseinat in bezug auf Fettemulgierung und Erhöhung der Viskosität einer Wurstemulsion und führt zu einem festeren Produkt
4	A. E. POARCH u. E. GWOZDZ US-PS 3 050 400 21. Aug. 1962 Western Dairy Products	*Magermilchpulver* (trocken) — mit verringertem Calciumgehalt auf 20 bis 70% des Normalgehaltes — konzentriert auf 30 bis 35% Feststoffgehalt — Sprühtrocknung	— Brühwurst — Zusatz von 0 ... 3,5%	— Verringerung des Fettabsatzes — Lactosegehalt → positive Beeinflussung des Flavors — Nährwert, Textur und Zartheit des Produktes verbessert — Schutzkolloideigenschaften
5	E. J. RIVOCHE US-PS 3 073 705 15. Jan. 1963 Rivark Research and Development Corporation	*Methylcellulose* und nichtionische Alkylether der Cellulose — Viskositätsgerade von 10 bis 15000 cp (in 2% wäßr. Lsg., bei 20 °C)	— Wurstprodukte, z. B. Frankfurter — eingesetzte Konzentrationen von 0,5 bis 5% in Abhängigkeit von der Viskosität der Cellulose — z. B. 1,5% Methocel mit 8000 cp Viskosität und 2% Methocel mit 4000 cp Viskosität	— Emulsionsstabilität erhöht — Schwund bei Herstellung verringert — besser gelöst durch Mischen mit wasserlöslichen Trockenmilchprodukten oder in heißem Wasser (> 85 °C) — Zugabe von Salz erniedrigt die Geltemperatur, die Gelbildung findet dann beim Kochen und Räuchern früher statt

Nr.	Autor Patent	Zusatzstoff bzw. -stoffgemisch	Einsatz (Menge und Produkt)	Bemerkung
6	J. A. MEUSEL R. A. BRUNN US-PS 3 148 071 8. Sept. 1964 Baltimore Spice Company	*Wärmebehandelte gemahlene Senfkörner* — Senfsamen enthalten u. a.: 27—38 % gebundenes Öl und das Enzym Myrosin, welches durch Wärmebehandlung zerstört wird	— Wurstprodukte, Brühwurst — 2 % ganze oder gemahlene Senfkörner, bezogen auf die Fleischmenge	— die in den Samen vorhandene Schleimsubstanz begünstigt das Schälen von Würsten in Darmhüllen — Samenproteine können den Geleeabsatz durch Absorptionseigenschaften vermindern — durch Wärmebehandlung (z. B. 1 ... 10 min; 110 ... 180 °C) Umwandlung des scharfen Senfgeschmacks in nußartigen milden Geschmack unter Erhaltung gewünschter physikalischer Eigenschaften
7	C. B. RASSMUSSEN US-PS 3 151 988 6. Okt. 1964 Stange Company	*Gemahlene, nichtrehydratisierte Senfkörner* — Partikelgröße 25 bis 200 Micron	— Wurstprodukte, z. B. Wurst aus Schweinefleisch mit einem 1 bis 2 %igen Zusatz	— Verringerung des Gewichtsverlustes während des Räucherns — Verringerung des Fettabsatzes, Emulsionsverbesserung, oxydativer Verderb (Fett) eingeschränkt, Farberhaltung, Verhinderung der Phasentrennung
8	A. E. POARCH US-PS 3 179 521 20. April 1965 Western Dairy Products	*Alkali-behandeltes Magermilchpulver* — Verwendung von Na- oder K-hydroxid oder Salzen von Alkalimetallen mit Phosphorsäure — pH-Einstellung auf 7,0 ... 7,3	— Wurstprodukte	— Verringerung des Fettabsatzes (außen) — verhindert die Bildung von sogen. „Fettnestern" im Wurstinneren
9	H. J. FETTY US-PS 3 216 827 9. 11. 1965	*Binder auf der Basis von Weizenmehl* Zusammensetzung — Gewichtsanteil (Beispiel) [%]	— Wurstprodukte, z. B. Bologner 3 ... 6 %iger Zusatz, auf Masse des Fleisches bezogen	— Verringerung des Fettabsatzes — Senkung der Gewichtsverluste — CO_2-Bildung und Ausbreitung im Fleisch, Verminderung der Fett- und Wasserverluste

		— Dicalciumphosphat-dihydrat — Natriumbicarbonat — Strukturiertes Füllmaterial, z. B. Weizenmehl oder entfettete Milchtrockenmasse — evtl. Geschmacksverstärker, z. B. hydrolysierte Pflanzenproteine, Mononatriumglutamat	45,3 15,1 10,7 1,0		
10	R. L. HELMER u. W. L. BROWN US-PS- 3 309 204 14. März 1967 John Morrell & Co.	*Pflanzliches Öl* z. B. Soja-Öl		— Wurstprodukte, z. B. Frankfurter 3 ... 30 % Zusatz 10 % bevorzugt	— erhöhte Emulsionsstabilität — Fettabsatz an Oberfläche und im Innern verringert — tierisches Fett zeigt nicht diese Effekte
11	H. E. WISTREICH H. J. GORSICA u. D. B. PERYAM US-PS 3 399 065 27. Aug. 1968 B. Heller & Co.	*entfettete Milchtrockenmasse mit Enzymzusatz* — Milchprotein (Casein) in situ (zerkl. Fleisch) durch Enzymwirkung präzipitiert — Enzymkonzentration (z. B. Rennin) 0,04 ... 0,1 % der Milchtrockenmasse		— Wurstprodukte — 1 ... 7 % Zusatz — 2,5 ... 4,5 % bevorzugt, über 7 % Geschmacksabweichungen des Produkts (Koch-Milch-Flavor) — günstig: Zugabe von Enzym und Milchprotein in Pulverform	— verbessert Wasserabsorption und Emulsionsstabilität — Binder
12	S. LIPNER US-PS 3 449 124 10. Juni 1969 Isolated Beef Protein Supplements Inc.	*Rinderblutplasmakonzentrat mit EDTA* Zugabe: — (0,1 ± 0,02) % Dinatrium-EDTA — 0,08 ... 0,1 % Dinatrium-EDTA bevorzugt (bezogen auf die eingesetzte Masse des Blutes) — Plasma, sprühgetrocknet bis 1,8 % Wassergehalt		— Wurstprodukte, z. B. Wiener, Frankfurter — 0,06 % ... 0,25 % Zusatz, bezogen auf die Fleischemulsion	— Binder für Fleischemulsionen — Nährwerterhöhung — Dinatriumsalz von EDTA wird dem frisch erschlachteten Blut zur Verhinderung der Koagulation zugesetzt

Nr.	Autor Patent	Zusatzstoff bzw. -stoffgemisch	Einsatz (Menge und Produkt)	Bemerkung
13	J. DAVID u. R. J. BERHOLD US-PS 3 469 995 30. Sept. 1969 Adolph's Food Products Mfg. Co., Burbank, California	*3 Zusatzstoffe und/oder deren Kombinationen* — *unmodifizierte Stärke* mit Anteil ≧ 50% Amylopectin, wie Weizenstärke, Getreidestärke, wachsige Reisstärke, Mais- und Sorghumstärke — *Chelatbildner*, z. B. mono- und dibasisches Natriumphosphat, Polyphosphate u. a. bevorzugt Natriumtripolyphosphat — *Protease* z. B. Chymotrypsin, Trypsin, Cathepsin, Pepsin u. a. bevorzugt Papain (Aktivität 3,9 bis 7,8 mg Tyrosin/100 ml)	— Produkte aus zerkleinertem Fleisch, z. B. Hamburger, Hackbraten — Einsatz von einem oder allen 3 Zusatzstoffen in Kombination zugesetzte Gewichtsanteile: *Chelatbildner*: 1 bis 7 Teile *unmodifizierte Wachsmaisstärke*: 1 bis 7 Teile *Protease*: 0,0004 bis 0,004 Teile	— Verbesserung von Wasserbindung und Textur — Senkung der Schwundverluste — die Kombination der 3 Zusatzstoffe ergibt eine stärkere Erhöhung der Wasserbindung als der Einsatz von zwei oder nur einem dieser Stoffe — Verbesserung der sensorischen Eigenschaften — zusätzlich ist die Zugabe von Farb- und Aromastoffen möglich
14	P. A. INKLAAR US-PS 3 617 307 2. Nov. 1971 Vasco Industries New York, N.Y.	*Protein-Aminosäuregemisch* — *wasserlösliches Protein* (z. B. Sojabohnen-, Milch- oder Eiprotein) — *α-Aminosäuren* von definierter Beschaffenheit und ein *pulverförmiger Puffer* (z. B. eine Mischung aus Natrium-Glycinat und Glycin oder Lysin-HCl, Histidin oder Methionin oder einem ihrer Salze u. a.)	— Hackfleisch-, Wurstprodukte, z. B. Hamburger, Frankfurter, Hackbraten, solche Produkte, die während der Herstellung wärmebehandelt werden — α-Aminosäurezusatz von 0,1 bis 1%, bezogen auf den Fleischgehalt der Wurstmasse — Zugabe zu Beginn bzw. während des Kutterprozesses, bevorzugt separate Zugabe der einzelnen Stoffe — Zugabemenge: • bis zu 6% wasserlösliches Protein (bezogen auf Gesamtmasse des Fleischproduktes)	— Proteinzusätze mit hohem NSI bevorzugt (40—100% wasserlöslich) — Fett- und Geleeabsatz verringert, insbesondere bei kombinierter Zugabe von Protein und α-Aminosäuren, synergistischer Effekt — Haltbarkeit verbessert — die Pufferkapazität einer 1%igen wäßrigen Lösung ist so groß, daß pro Gramm des Gemisches mehr als 20 ml 0,1 N Säure zur pH-Verschiebung von 10 auf 6 benötigt werden.

			• Protein-Aminosäuregemisch: 10 bis 98 Teile wasserlösliches Protein, 1 bis 10 Teile bestimmter Aminosäuren	
15	St. LIPNER US-PS 3 644 128 22. Febr. 1972	*Blutplasma-Hydrokolloid-Binder* Zusammensetzung des Binders: — 0,01 bis 0,5 bzw. 0,0625 % Extrakt eines wasserlöslichen Hydrokolloids, z. B. sulfatierte Polysaccharide, Carrageenan — 99,5 bis 99,9 % eines getrockneten Plasmaprotein-Anteils von tierischem Blut	— Produkte aus zerkleinertem Fleisch, z. B. Frankfurter, Bologner — Binder-Zusatz 0,04 bis 5,0 %, bezogen auf die Gesamtmasse des Produkts — Zugabe in Form eines sprühgetrockneten Pulvers	— Textur- und Nährwertverbesserung zum Herstellen einer Kaltemulsion
16	B. J. CATLIN und T. B. WILLIAMS DE-EB 2 421 541 28. Nov. 1974 Unilever N.v., Rotterdam	*Kartoffelprodukt* — getrocknete Kartoffelpulpe, die Zellwandpolysaccharide und Stärke im Verhältnis von wenigstens 1:1 enthält	— für getrocknete Produkte aus zerkleinertem Fleisch und Gemische aus Fleisch und texturierten Pflanzenproteinen geeignet — Zugabemengen zwischen 1 und 10 %, bezogen auf das Naßgewicht des zerkleinerten Fleisches	— zur Herstellung eines leicht rehydratisierbaren getrockneten Fleischproduktes geeignet
17	A. A. SCHULZ US-PS 3 900 576 19. Aug. 1975 Miles Laboratories, Elkhart, Ind.	*Zusatzstoffgemisch (Extender)* zusammengesetzt aus: a) 39 bis 48,5 % Pflanzenproteinfasern b) 5,5 bis 12 % Pflanzenproteinisolat c) 2 bis 5 % Eiweiß (Eiklar) d) 0 bis 6 % Pflanzenproteinkonzentrat e) 4,5 bis 5,5 % Molke f) 0,1 bis 1,5 % Emulgator g) 1 bis 5 % Milchtrockenmasse h) 9 bis 18 % Gluten (oder Mischung von Mehl und Wasser) i) 0 bis 1,5 % Salz j) 15,5 bis 19 % Wasser — bezogen auf die Gesamtmasse des Gemisches	— geeignet für Fleischemulsionen, z. B. Frankfurter, Geflügel- oder Fischprodukte — 30 bis 70 % Extender werden dem Fleischbrät zugegeben	— Emulsionsstabilität verbessert, auch nach der Wärmebehandlung — Zusatz von Gewürzen (0,05 bis 1 %), Vitaminen und Mineralstoffen möglich

Nr.	Autor Patent	Zusatzstoff bzw. -stoffgemisch	Einsatz (Menge und Produkt)	Bemerkung
18	L. V. NAGEL US-PS 3 914 457 21. Okt. 1975	— getrocknetes *Sojaproteinextrudat* wird mit heißem, 0,1 % Gewürze enthaltendem Wasser gequollen und mit zerkleinerten *tierischen Proteinen gemischt* — Anteil des Sojaproteins beträgt 20 bis 29 % am Gesamtprotein des Produkts — Verwendung *weiterer Zusatzstoffe* möglich (z. B. Emulgatoren, Tenderizer u. a.)	— Produkte aus zerkleinertem Fleisch oder Fisch — Verhältnis: heißes Wasser : Soja-extrudat : tierisches Protein 1 : 1 : 3 15 : 5 : 1	— zwischen Produkten mit und ohne Zusatzstoff besteht sensorisch kein Unterschied
19	A. E. HAWKINS DE-OS 2 522 786 11. Dez. 1975 Unilever N.V., Rotterdam	*Proteinhaltige Materialien* aus: — globulären u./o. myofibrillären Proteinen oder — Sojaproteinen (25—30 % Protein) 2—5 % NaCl, pH 4,8—5,4 durch Zusatz zu einem strömenden Koaguliermedium entsteht ein Produkt mit einem mindestens *10fach vergrößerten Oberflächenbereich* — Schichtdicke ≦ 100 μ. — Länge 10 bis 30 mm	— Einsatz in fleischähnlichen Produkten, Fleischanalogen und -semianalogen — zu rekonstituiertem Fleisch	— durch große Oberfläche stark wasserbindend — strukturbildend bei Fleischanalogen — Verfahren zur Herstellung dieser Materialien beschrieben
20	N. W. DESROSIER DE-OS 2 617 260 27. Okt. 1977 Plymouth, Mass.	*Streckungsmittel* aus — zu Flocken verarbeiteten Weizenkernen mit und ohne Kleie, gemischt mit einer Fleischaromasubstanz — Zusatz von Protein-, Vitamin- und Mineralsalzergänzungssubstanzen sowie Antipilzmitteln	— Hackfleischprodukte aus Rind-, Schweine-, Schaf- und Geflügelfleisch, Innereien, Fischfleisch u. a. tierischen Gewebe	— Verfahren zur Herstellung beschrieben

21	F. EPSTEIN u. P. R. EPSTEIN US-PS 4 123 557 31. Okt. 1978 Long Island City, N.Y.	*Binder auf Milchprotein-Lactose-Basis* a) Milchproteine: Albumin und Casein im Verhältnis 14—24:7—20 bzw. 1:1 b) Lactose Verhältnis Lactose zu Protein 38—50:28—35 (Gewichtsanteile) bzw. 3:2	— Produkte aus zerkleinertem Fleisch (Frankfurter, Bologner, Frühstücksfleisch) — Zugabemenge z. B. 4%, bez. auf Gesamtmasse des Produkts	— verbesserte Bindung, die den Bindungseigenschaften des undenaturierten Myosins entspricht
22	W. M. LINDL u. a. US-PS 4 071 635 31. Jan. 1978 General Mills Inc., USA	*Stoffgemisch aus:* % a) Stärke o. stärkehalt. Mat. (z. B. modifizierte Getreidestärke, Tapiocastärke) 25 bis 85 b) Proteinkomponente (z. B. Eialbumin und Sojaisolat im Verhältnis 48:1 bis 1:48) 1,5 bis 55 c) Fleischpökelstoff (z. B. Natriumnitrit) 0,1 bis 3,0 d) Polyphosphat 0,1 bis 15,0 e) Natriumchlorid 1,0 bis 25,0 f) Pflanzenöl 0 bis 15,0 g) Säuerungsmittel 0 bis 25,0 h) Aromastoffe, Gewürze, Farbstoffe 0 bis 25,0	— Produkte aus zerkleinertem Fleisch — Zusatz von Wasser: Trockengemisch 1,5 bis 4:1 — Verhältnis: zerkl. Fleisch : Stoffgemisch-Wasserkomb. 1 : 0,25 bis 1 : 2,5	— Kochverlust verringert — Backen und Kochen der Produkte möglich
23	N. MELACHOURIS DE-OS 2 900-442 19. Juli 1979 Staufer Chemical Co., Westport, Conn.	*Modifizierter Molkenfeststoff* enthält: 23 bis 54 Gew.-% Lactose 24 bis 60 Gew.-% Mineralstoffe 15 bis 27 Gew.-% Protein	— zum Strecken von zerkleinerten Fleischprodukten — max. 3,5 Gew.-% Zusatz zu Wurst und 10 bis 20 Gew.-% zu Hackfleischerzeugnissen — als trockenes Pulver zugesetzt	— Molkenfeststoffe als Ausfällung erhalten, beim Zusatz eines zweiwertigen Metallions zu einer Käsemolkenlösung und pH-Einstellung zwischen 6 und 8 — die Käsemolkenlösung kann

Nr.	Autor Patent	Zusatzstoff bzw. -stoffgemisch	Einsatz (Menge und Produkt)	Bemerkung
				20, 60 oder 100% saure Molke enthalten — Streckung und Geschmacksstabilisierung der Produkte — verbesserte Wasserbindung und Fettemulgierung
24	S. WENZEL u. B. RÖTTGER DE-OS 2 816 865 25. Okt. 1979 Hannover	*aufgeschlossenes Bluteiweiß aus Chromoproteiden* — Abtrennung der Globineiweißkomponente aus Blut bzw. Chromoproteiden durch Hämolyse — pH-Wert des Globineiweißes auf 5,4 bis 6,6 eingestellt — pH = 5,8 ... 6,2 bevorzugt	Wurstprodukte, z. B. Lyoner — Zugabe in einer Lösung oder in getrockneter Form — 0,2 bis 5% aufgeschl. Bluteiweiß (berechnet als Trockengewicht u. bezogen auf Brätmasse) — 0,5 bis 2,5% günstige, — 0,8 bis 1,5% bevorzugte Zugabemenge	— Eiweißgehalt erhöht — Geschmack, Konsistenz u. Haltbarkeit verbessert — Emulgier- und Wasserbindungsfähigkeit verbessert
25	M. SHEMER US-PS 4 188 399 12. Feb. 1980 Miles Laboratories, Inc.	*viskoses wärmekoagulierbares Protein aus Ölsamen* — Herstellung: in einer 8 bis 12%igen wäßrigen Lsg. wird ein pH von 5,1 bis 5,9 (bevorzugt pH 5,5) eingestellt — nach Extraktion der säurelöslichen Proteine (bei ca. 40 °C, Rühren) werden der flüssige Anteil der Aufschwemmung vom unlöslichen abgetrennt (Filtration o. Zentrifugieren) und die Proteine durch isoelektr. Fällung, Ultrafiltration, Umkehrosmose u. a. m. gewonnen	— Emulgator, Binder insbesondere für Fleischanaloga	— Protein mit guten funktionellen und Wärmekoagulations-Eigenschaften — Herstellungsprozeß beschrieben — Zugabe von Antioxydantien zur Extraktionslösung nötig (bevorzugt 0,1 bis 1 Gew.-% Natriumsulfit, bezogen auf das Gewicht der Ölsäuren)
26	A. E. POARCH US-PS 4 202 907	*enzymaktiviertes Natriumcaseinat* — durch Kationenaustausch wird	— zerkleinerte Fleischprodukte, Wurst	— bildet bei der Wärmebehandlung (in Brühwurst) ein festes

	13. Mai 1980	Calciumphosphocaseinat zu Natriumcaseinat umgewandelt — Labenzym zugesetzt	— Zugabemenge 3,5 bis 20%, bezogen auf das Endgewicht der Wurst	nichtreversibles Gel, das auch beim Kühlen stabil bleibt — Gelbildung tritt bei einem Calciumgehalt von 8 bis 70 mg/100 ml auf (bevorzugt = 8 mg/100 ml)
27	E. SCHIFFNER, E. SCHARNER u. G. PETTER DD-WP 0 152 470 3. Juni 1980	*Molkenkonzentrat* — nicht hitzedenaturiert — mit Speisesalzzusatz bis a_w < 0,87 (100 l Molkenkonzentrat + 10 kg Speisesalz) — zu 100 l Molkenkonzentrat Zusatz von 3 kg Polyphosphat — Zusatz d. Starterflüssigkultur des Stammes SSHK 76 zum Molkenkonzentrat oder zur Brühwurstmasse	— Brühwurst, z. B. Bockwurst — Zusatzmenge: z. B. 8 l Molkenkonzentrat auf 40 kg Fleisch (S 2 u. S 3)	— Qualitätsverbesserung, Erhöhung der Wasserbindung, Verbesserung der ernährungsphysiol. Wertigkeit, materialökonomischer Effekt — Kerntemperatur beim Brühen muß 80 °C erreichen (Koagulation d. β-Lactoglobulins)
28	E. SCHIFFNER, E. SCHARNER u. K. SIEBERT DD-WP 0 152 471 3. Juni 1980	*Säuregefälltes Casein* — Säurefällung d. Caseins aus Magermilch durch Zusatz des Kokkenkonzentrates d. Stammes SSHK 76 u. a. Mikroorganismenkulturen	— Brühwürste — Zusatzmenge d. Caseins 10%, bezogen auf die Brätmasse — Zugabe am Ende des Kutterprozesses	— Qualitätsverbesserung, Verbesserung der Materialökonomie — Verbesserung von Konsistenz und Umrötung — 3/5 des zugesetzten Nitritpökelsalzes werden durch Steinsalz ersetzt
29	R. HANSEN u. a. DD-WP 151 688 30. Juni 1980	*Fremdproteinkonzentrat(gemisch)* aus: — 70 Gew.-% thermostabilem Milcheiweißpräzipitat und 30 Gew.-% thermokoabulierbarem Proteinkonzentrat (Eialbumin, natives Molkenproteinkonzentrat, Blutproteine sowie primäre Proteine, einzeln oder in Kombination) oder — 100 Gew.-% thermostabilem Milcheiweißkopräzipitat	— Zusatz zu zerkleinertem Rohfleisch aller Schlachttiere und Fische — Zusatz trocken in Pulverform oder mit Wasser angeteigt von 5 bis 95 Gew.-%, bevorzugt 5 bis 30 Gew.-%	— kaubare Gele und Fasern gebildet — hohes Wasserbindungsvermögen der Fremdproteine — ökonomisch und technologisch vorteilhaft

Nr.	Autor Patent	Zusatzstoff bzw. -stoffgemisch	Einsatz (Menge und Produkt)	Bemerkung
30	D. J. PHILLIPS D. T. JONES u. D. E. PALMER US-PS 4 218 490 19. Aug. 1980 Viscose Group Limited, Croydon, England	*Funktionelles Protein* — gewonnen durch Extraktion bzw. Ionenaustausch aus folgenden Quellen: Blut, Soja, Eiklar, Milch, Rapssamen u. a. — konzentriert durch Ultrafiltration — Gel gebildet (T, p, pH, Konz.) und evtl. getrocknet	— als Schaumbildner in Baisermassen, Marshmallows, Makronengebäcken u. a. — Wasserbindung u. Fettemulgierung in Wurstprodukten — einsetzbar in zerkleinerten Fleisch-, Fisch- und Gemüseprodukten und in Getränken, in Gelform oder getrocknet	— mit wenigstens einer der folgenden Eigenschaften: schaumbildend oder -stabilisierend, wasserbindend, fettemulgierend und gelbildend
31	M. SHEMER US-PS 4 238 515 9. Dez. 1980 Development Co. Ltd., Israel	*Gluten-Pflanzenprotein-Binder* — an die Glutenmatrix ist ein inerter Feststoff mit einer Partikelgröße < 5 cm ∅ (texturiertes Pflanzenprotein bzw. rehydratisiertes extrudiertes Sojaeiweiß) gebunden — Gluten mit einer netzähnlichen Faserstruktur, Faserdurchmesser < 2 mm u. Viskosität ≧ 50000 cps	— Fleischanaloga — Fleisch- und Wurstprodukte, z. B. Hamburger, Cornedbeef — weitere Einsatzmöglichkeiten bei der Papier-, Klebstoff-, Puddingherstellung	— gute Bindungseigenschaften, Texturverbesserung und verbesserte Wasserbindung im Produkt, Ersatzstoff für Eiklar — *Herstellung:* Weizenvitalgluten wird mit einem Reduktionsmittel (Tocopherol, Ascorbinsäure, Natriumsulfit) bei T < 70 °C behandelt u. gleichzeitig der inerte Lebensmittelfeststoff (∅ < 5 cm) im Verhältnis 1:0,1 bis 1:10 (Gluten: Feststoff) zugegeben
32	R. M. LAUCK und N. MELACHOURIS US-PS 4 259 363 31. März 1981 Stauffer Chemical Company	*Molken-Caseinat-Binder-Gemisch* 5 bis 50 Gew.-% Casein oder dessen Natrium- und Kaliumsalze gemischt mit 5 bis 50 Gew.-% Molkenfeststoffen mit verringertem Lactose- oder Proteingehalt (Permeat, UF) und getroeknet	— Produkte aus zerkleinertem Fleisch, Schmorfleisch, Suppen, Bratensoße, Paniermehl, Teig, Käseprodukten u. a. — Zugabe 1 bis 35%	— das Zusatzstoffgemisch kann als Aromaverstärker, Aromastoff oder Binder eingesetzt werden — Herstellungsprozeß beschrieben — Wasserbindung stabilisiert

33	T. V. NGUYEN und T. J. WAGNER US-PS 4 276 319 30. Jun. 1981 Ralstron Purina Company, St. Louis	*Granuliertes Protein-Gel* — Pflanzenproteinisolat (Sojaproteinisolat) mit einem Eiweißgehalt ≧ 90 Gew.-% u. guten Gelbildungseigenschaften (Viskosität beträgt bei 25 °C 0,9 bis 1,1 × 10^6 cps) — das Isolat wird hydratisiert, granuliert und getrocknet	— Extender für Fleischprodukte	— das granulierte und getrocknete Proteinprodukt besitzt ein ausgezeichnetes Rehydratationsvermögen — Wasseraufnahmevermögen ≧ 4 g/g Granulat — Herstellungsprozeß: Gemisch Pflanzenproteinisolat u. 60 bis 75% (65 bis 70%) Wasser werden bei 75 °C bis 125 °C (80°—100 °C) extrudiert, granuliert und getrocknet (z. B. luftgetrocknet zwischen 87 und 98 °C)
34	C. J. LYNCH, C. F. LIN u. N. MELACHOURIS EP 0 046 639 3. März 1982 Stauffer Chemical Company, Westport Connecticut, entspricht US-PS 4 348 420 7. Sept. 1982	*Binder* bestehend aus a + b: a) 99,5 bis 50% eines wasserlöslichen *proteinhaltigen Stoffes*: z. B. Natrium- und Kaliumcaseinat, Molkenproteinkonzentrat und deren Gemische, Blut- und Fleischeiweiße sowie *Nebenprodukte* aus der Gelfiltration der *Molke* u. das Permeat bzw. das laktosefreie Permeat der ultrafiltrierten Molke b) 0,5 bis 50% eines *Hydrokolloids* z. B. Alginat, Carrageenan, Guarkernmehl, Gummi arabicum, Johannisbrotkernmehl, Carboxylmethylcellulose und Carboxylmethylstärke	— Produkte aus zerkleinertem Fleisch, z. B. Wurstprodukte, Hackbraten; mit 1 bis 15 Gew.-% Binderzusatz, bezogen auf Masse Fleisch u. Binder (ungekocht) a) *bevorzugt*: Natriumcaseinat u. laktosefreies Permeat im Verhältnis 75:25 bis 25:75 b) *bevorzugt*: 1 bis 10% Anteil des Hydrokolloids im Binder; 0,01 bis 4% Anteil des Hydrokolloids im ungekochten Fleischprodukt (Fleisch + Binder)	— verbesserte Bindungseigenschaften — bevorzugtes Bindergemisch: wasserlösliches Protein/Hydrokolloid/Nebenprodukt aus Molke
35	E. CONRAD EP 0 049 695 14. April 1982 Maslin AB Plavia, Stockholm	*Austauschstoff* enthält: a) die *Gluten-Protein- und* die *Kleie-Fraktion* von Getreidekörnern bzw. *Weizenkörnern* b) die *Hämoglobinfraktion* von	— Produkte aus zerkleinertem Fleisch — Substitutionsgrad bis zu 50 Gew.-% TM, bezogen auf den Fleischgehalt — der Gluten-Kleie-Anteil im	— Nährwertverbesserung, Aminosäurezusammensetzung verändert — Kosten gesenkt — Herstellungsprozeß für Austauschstoff beschrieben

Nr.	Autor Patent	Zusatzstoff bzw. -stoffgemisch	Einsatz (Menge und Produkt)	Bemerkung
		Schlachttierblut bis zu 15 Gew.-%, bezogen auf das TM-Gewicht der Gluten-Kleie-Fraktion (bevorzugt 4 bis 6 Gew.-%) c) ein *Milchprodukt* in Form von *Käse-Schaum* mit einem Anteil bis zu 40 Gew.-% TM (bevorzugt 20 bis 35 Gew.-%), bezogen auf das TM-Gewicht der Gluten-Kleie-Fraktion	Fleischprodukt beträgt 10 bis 25 Gew.-% TM	
36	G. W. P. Bams u. J. Visser EP 0 051 423 12. Mai 1982 Unilever N.V.	— texturiertes *caseinhaltiges Material* — extrudierte Masse aus Wasser und proteinhaltigem Material mit ≧ 60 Gew.-% Casein oder Caseinaten, pflanzlichen oder tierischen Proteinisolaten u./o. -konzentraten, Magermilchpulver und Gluten	— Extender für Fleisch- oder Fischprodukte — Fleisch- o. Fischanaloga	
37	J. A. Ederle, R. A. Hoer u. G. H. Irwin US-PS 4 391 840 5. Juli 1983	*Proteinextender mit TiO_2-Tracer* — Gemisch aus Pflanzenproteinisolat u. TiO_2 wird hydratisiert bis zu 40 bis 75% Wassergehalt (pH d. Lsg. 4,3 bis 4,8) — behandelt bei Temp. 148 °C bis 157 °C — eine unlösl. Matrix gebildet — die Matrix wird in Form kleiner getrockneter Partikel mit einem Pflanzenprotein gemischt, hydratisiert und extrudiert	— Fleischprodukte	— Nährwert beeinflußt — unerwünschte Farbabweichungen vermieden — Herstellungsprozeß beschrieben
38	P. J. Senior u. J. Mc Nairney	— *Einzellerprotein* (SCP) bakterieller Herkunft	— Produkte aus zerkleinertem Fleisch oder Fisch	— positiver Einfluß auf Textur und Geschmack des Produkts

	EP 0 088 530 14. Sept. 1983 Imperial Chemical Industries PLC, G.B.	— bevorzugt von Methylophilus methylotrophus — *sowie Pflanzenöl* — SCP mit durchschnittlicher Partikelgröße von 40 bis 500 μ	— Zugabe von SCP in Pulverform in Mengen von 0,5 bis 15%; zu funktionellen Zwecken von 0,5 bis 2%	
39	R. WINTER DE-OS 3 221 143 A 1 27. Okt. 1983 Fa. FIBA, R. Winter	*Gelee-Emulsion* aus: E 471 Mono- und Diglyceriden v. Speisefettsäuren E 472 b Mono- und Diglyceriden v. Speisefettsäuren verestert mit Milchsäure E 472 c Mono- u. Diglyceriden v. Speisefettsäuren verestert mit Citronensäure E 331 Trinatriumcitrat Stabilisator: Tierisches Eiweiß mit NaCl	— Wurstprodukte — Zusatz 5—10%, bezogen auf Masse des Magerfleisches — Zugabe erfolgt in Gelee-Form	— geeignet zur Herstellung eines bei hohen Temperaturen stabilen Brätes ohne Gelee- oder Fettabsatz — Tierisches Eiweiß wird nicht näher benannt.
40	L. WALLINGFORD u. T. P. LABUZA, 1983	*Hydrokolloide* — Xanthan — Carrageenan — Pektin (niedrig verestert) — Johannisbrotgummi	Modellbrät (geringer Fettgehalt, 11% Proteingehalt) mit 0,2 Gew.-% Hydrokolloidzusatz (bezogen auf Gesamtmasse des Brätansatzes)	g Wasserverlust (Kochverlust) pro 100 g ungekochtes Modellbrät Xanthan 2,91 ± 0,85 Carrageenan 3,99 ± 1,08 Johannisbrotgummi 8,39 ± 3,26 Pektin (niedrig verestert) 20,05 ± 1,85 — die Untersuchungen am Modellbrät waren mit denen an der Baumann-Apparatur gemessenen Wasseraufnahmemengen (für die Hydrokolloide) vergleichbar
41	E. PUOLANNE u. M. RUUSUMEN 1983	*Kartoffelmehl und Milchpulver*	Modellbrät aus Rind- und Schweinefleisch — Zugabe von Kartoffelmehl u. Milchpulver einzeln und in Kombination	— bis zu einem Kartoffelmehlgehalt von 6% stieg das Wasserbindungsvermögen (WBV) des Brühwurstmodellbrätes stark an und blieb dann nahezu konstant (bis 10%)

Nr.	Autor Patent	Zusatzstoff bzw. -stoffgemisch	Einsatz (Menge und Produkt)	Bemerkung
			— Einsatzmenge 0 bis 10%, bezogen auf die Masse des Grundbrätes	— gleichzeitige Milchpulverzugabe verbessert das WBV nur bei kleinen Zugabemengen an Kartoffelmehl — Milchpulverzugabe von 2 bis 4% führte zu einer WBV-Steigerung, bei gleichzeitigem Kartoffelmehlzusatz war die Steigerung geringer
42	A. S. BAWA Diss. Kanada 1984	*Zusatzstoffe u. Gemische* Weizenmehl, Promax-70, Natriumcaseinat, Getreidestärke, Magermilchpulver, Senfmehl	Produkte aus zerkleinertem Fleisch, 3 Modellsysteme (stark, mittel, schwach)	— die Zusatzstoffe (Extender, Filler) wirken antagonistisch im starken und synergistisch im mittleren und schwachen System — Wiener mit Natriumcaseinat-Zugabe erreichten die höchsten Punktzahlen hinsichtlich sensorischer Qualität
43	J. SHIRO KUDO u. S. M. MUKAIYAMA US-PS 4 504 514 12. März 1985 Takeda Chemical Ind. Ltd. Japan	*faserförmiges oder granuliertes Produkt auf Soja-Basis* — unter Verwendung von organ. Säure (2 bis 6 C-Atome) und/oder Metallkationen in Form eines eßbaren Salzes (Calciumchlorid, -sulfat, Magnesiumsalz) — 0,03 bis 0,6 g Ca-, Mg-Salz pro kg Soja-Material — Sojamaterial gemahlen mit einem Wassergehalt von 30—60 Gew.-% und 0,01 bis 2 g Essigsäure/kg	— Zusatzstoff für Produkte aus zerkleinertem Fleisch und Fisch	— Produkte mit Zusatzstoff besitzen eine verbesserte Textur

44	T. TSUCHIYA Jap.-PS 60 248 153 22. Mai 1985	— *Proteinpulver* oder *-lösung* aus: 33 ... 65% Sojaprotein 22 ... 54% Lactalbumin 9 ... 28% Albumin 4 ... 20% Serumprotein — Serumprotein, bevorzugt gewonnen aus zentrifugiertem und sprühgetrocknetem Tierblut	— Fleisch- oder Fischprodukte werden mit dem Proteingemisch imprägniert bzw. sie adsorbieren es	— Produkte mit guter Farbe und Textur erhalten — Wasserverlust verhindert
45	G. MIETH u. CH. SCHNEIDER DD-WP 223 355 12. Juni 1985 AdW der DDR	— *strukturiertes Protein* aus pflanzlichen, tierischen und/oder mikrobiellen Rohstoffen, vorzugsweise Proteinisolaten	— Fleisch- oder Fischprodukte und in küchenfertiger Speisenzubereitung — Zugabe z. B.: 20 Gew.-% strukturiertes Protein (z. B. Casein) 70 Gew.-% zerkleinertes Rindfleisch 10 Gew.-% Schmalz	— hohe Wasser- und Fettbindung bei unterschiedlichen pH-Werten
46	E. RAUTILA Finnland DE-EB 3 444 642 5. Sept. 1985	— *Gemisch* aus Milchpulver, Kartoffelmehl und Wasser — als sogen. flüssiger „Schlamm" in ständiger Bewegung gehalten, gut dosierbar, homogen	— Produkte aus zerkleinertem Fisch — Zugabe: Dosierung wird entsprechend der Rezeptur automatisch gesteuert	— Mischen, Steuern und Dosieren beschrieben
47	E. M. KÖHLER u. a. DD-WP 227 876 2. Okt. 1985	— Lebensmittelzusatzprodukt aus *Biertreber* und *Getreidemahlprodukt* — Verhältnisse von Biertreber: Getreidemahlprodukt 1 : 10 1 : 1 — aus Biertreber (60—90% Trebersaftgehalt) u. Getreidemahlprodukt eine Masse bereitet; diese extrudiert (T = 373 K, p = 10 bis 35 MPa) und vermahlen	— Zusatzstoff für Fleischerzeugnisse, Hackfleischmassen, Fisch- und Backwaren	— zur Herstellung kein großer apparativer Aufwand erforderlich — Zusatzstoff vielfältig einsetzbar — herkömmlicher Kneter, ein Extruder und eine Mahleinrichtung erforderlich
48	J. KROLL u. a. DD-WP 229 924	*cellulosehaltige Materialien* — aus einer Milchsäuregärung u/o.	— Herstellung von Fleischerzeugnissen, Wurst- u.	— Stabilisierung des Wasserbindungsvermögens und der

Nr.	Autor Patent	Zusatzstoff bzw. -stoffgemisch	Einsatz (Menge und Produkt)	Bemerkung
	20. Nov. 1985 AdW der DDR	einer Hypochloriteinwirkung unterworfenen lignocellulosehaltigen pflanzlichen Rohstoffen, vorzugsweise aus Blatt- u. Wurzelgemüse oder aus den Rückständen der industriellen Obst-, Gemüse- und Hackfruchtverarbeitung hergestellt	Hackfleischprodukten, Pasteten oder Fleischkonserven aus zerkleinertem und vermischtem Fleisch — Zugabemenge: 0,05 bis 2,0 TM-%, bevorzugt 0,1 bis 1,5 TM-%, bezogen auf den Fleischeinsatz — Zugabe der behandelten pflanzlichen Rohstoffe in feuchtem, emulgiertem, trockenem u/o. rehydriertem Zustand	Herstellung von Fleischerzeugnissen — Gemische werden einer Wärmebehandlung u/o. weiterer konservierender oder geschmacksgebender Behandlung unterworfen
49	W. E. SCHWARTZ u. a. US-P 4 556 571 3. Dez. 1985 Stauffer Chemical Companie, USA	— *Sojaprodukt* aus Sojamehl, -konzentrat, -isolat mit Proteingehalt von 40 bis 90% — mit *Hefelösung* (z. B. Saccharomyces cerevisiae) behandelt bis 100% d. Eigengewichts an Lösung aufgenommen werden	— Produkte aus zerkleinertem Fleisch	— verringerter Bohnengeschmack — Ausbeute konstant gehalten
50	J. KROLL u. H. PETERS DD WPA 23 L/300 033.1 19. Febr. 1987 AdW der DDR	*stärkehaltiger Zusatzstoff in Granulatform* aus: — stärkehaltigem Trägermaterial (z. B. Kartoffel-, Weizen-, Maisstärke, Getreidemehle o. -schrote) — Protein und/oder (aus proteinhaltigen Lösungen, wie Blutplasma, -serum, Molke, Magermilch, Pflanzenextrakte) — Aromastoffe und/oder Würzmittel Masseverhältnis von Stärke zu Protein vorzugsweise 70:30 bis 50:50	— Erzeugnisse aus zerkleinertem, wärmebehandeltem Fleisch oder Fisch	— Stabilisierung der Wasserbindung — Verbesserung der Ausbeute

wasser- bzw. emulsionsstabilisierende Eigenschaften von Zusatzstoffen zu bestimmen. Bei allen wird der Anspruch erhoben, den Praxisbedingungen am nächsten zu kommen.

Beispiele für Methoden zur Untersuchung von Zusätzen zu Fleisch- und Fleischerzeugnissen sind in Tab. 2 zusammengefaßt. Zur Charakterisierung der Einflüsse von Zusatzstoffen wenden zahlreiche Autoren die Kochverlustbestimmung sowie sensorische und rheologische Methoden an. Grundlegende Untersuchungen zur Charakterisierung der molekularen Wechselwirkungen zwischen Zusatzstoffen und Fleischproteinen sind relativ selten. Sie betreffen vorzugsweise Wechselwirkungen von Soja- bzw. Milchproteinfraktionen mit Myosin [4—12].

In Tab. 3 sind aus der Sicht der fleischverarbeitenden Industrie an die Zusatzstoffe bzw. -stoffgemische zu stellende Forderungen zusammengefaßt. Die funktionellen Eigenschaften sind entsprechend Tab. 1 einem bestimmten Zerkleinerungsgrad der Fleischprodukte zugeordnet. Ausführliche Überblicke über die funktionellen Eigenschaften einzelner „Fleisch"-Zusatzstoffe geben VISSER [2, 3], MANN [13], MITTAL u. a. [14], BAWA [15] sowie HOLLAND [16]. In Fortsetzung des Fortschrittsberichtes von KROLL u. a. [1] wird in Tab. 4 unter Auswertung der Patentliteratur ein Überblick über Zusatzstoffe bzw. deren Gemische gegeben, die verschiedenen Fleischsystemen in unterschiedlicher Form und Menge zugesetzt worden sind.

Schlußbemerkungen

In der Patentliteratur (siehe Tab. 4) wird eine Vielzahl von Stoffen genannt, die in Produkten aus zerkleinertem Fleisch auf Grund ihrer Eigenschaften zur Beeinflussung der Wasserbindung und Fettemulgierung (Kochverlust, Safthaltevermögen) beitragen sollen. Den Hauptanteil davon haben Zusatzstoffe bzw. Compounds auf der Basis von Milch-bzw. Molken- (vgl. [2]), Pflanzen- (vgl. [1]) und Blutproteinen, gefolgt von solchen auf Polysaccharidbasis (z. B. Stärke, Cellulose). Derartige Stoffe werden Fleischerzeugnissen einzeln oder in Kombination bzw. unter Zugabe von Enzymen, Hydrokolloiden, Phosphaten, Salzen und/oder Emulgatoren zugesetzt. Aus der Theorie der Strukturbildung thermisch behandelter Fleischerzeugnisse (z. B. Brühwürste) läßt sich ableiten, daß Zusatzstoffgemische dieser Art sowohl die Brät- als auch die Produktstruktur unterstützten sollen [17—20].

Nach OELKER [17] und SIEGEL u. a. [21] sollten die Compounds Bestandteile enthalten, die a) eine den Myofilamentfragmenten ähnliche Struktur und Dimensionierung besitzen; b) in den Zwischenräumen der myofilamentären Flockenstruktur z. B. gegarter Brühwurst Substrukturate ausbilden und c) hydrokolloidale Eigenschaften aufweisen, um das bei der Proteindenaturation freiwerdende Wasser aufnehmen zu können. Die in Vorschlag gebrachten Stoffgemische sind den Fleisch-/Modellsystemen überwiegend in Pulverform, und zwar als Texturate, Strukturate oder Gele zugesetzt worden. Die Zusatzgrenze scheint im Falle von Hackfleischmassen bei 20—25% zu liegen, sofern Texturate oder Strukturate eingebracht werden. Pulverförmige Compounds bzw. Zusatzstoffe können Produkten aus zerkleinertem Fleisch (speziell Brühwürsten) ohne sensorische Beeinträchtigung selten mehr als in Anteilen von 2 bis 5% zugegeben werden. Bei hochwirksamen bzw. funktionellen Zusätzen oder Compounds (z. B. Tab. 4, Nr. 48 und Nr. 50) sollen schon Beimengungen von 2 Gew.-% zu einer deutlichen Verbesserung der Wasserbindung und Fettemulgierung und damit zu einer Ausbeuteerhöhung führen.

Summary

H. PETERS, J. KROLL and B. GASSMANN: Studies on the application of additives and compounds in meat products

From the economic and perspective point of view the application of compounds and extenders in meat products represents an unavoidable world-wide development. The present study reviews additives and compounds for sausages and other comminuted meat products which have an influence on water binding and fat emulsifying. In the paper details and results of the patent publications published since 1960 are presented and discussed.

Резюме

Х. ПЕТЕРС, Й. КРОЛЛЬ и Б. ГАССМАНН: Использование добавочных веществ и смесей веществ (compounds) в мясных продуктах

С экономической точки зрения и точки зрения перспективного развития, использование смесей добавочных веществ (compounds) и разбавителей в мясных продуктах является неизбежным и касающимся всех стран развитием. Настоящий обзор дает представление о добавочных веществах или смесей веществ, которые добавляются к колбасным изделиям и другим продуктам из измельченного мяса с целью влияния на водосвязывание и эмульгирование жира. В этом смысле анализируется имеющаяся с 1960 года патентная литература.

Literatur

[1] KROLL, J., und B. GASSMANN, Nahrung **27**, 699 (1983).
[2] VISSER, F. M. W., in: Milk Proteins' 84. Herausgegeben von T. E. GALESLOOT und B. J. TINBERGEN. 206—216. Pudoc, Wageningen 1985.
[3] VISSER, F. M. W., in: Proceedings of IDF Symposium on Dairy Ingredients in the Food Industry. 42—46. IDF, Luxemburg 1981.
[4] HAGA, S., und T. OHASHI, Nippon Shokunin Kogyo Gakkaishi **25**, 226—231 (1978).
[5] HAGA, S., und T. OHASHI, Nippon Shokunin Kogyo Gakkaishi **26**, 429 (1979).
[6] HAGA, S., und T. OHASHI, Nippon Shokunin Kogyo Gakkaishi **27**, 433 (1980).
[7] HAGA, S., und T. OHASHI, Nippon Shokunin Kogyo Gakkaishi **28**, 189 (1981).
[8] PENG, I. C., W. R. DAYTON, D. W. QUASS, und C. E. ALLEN, J. Food Sci. **47**, 1976—1983, 1984—1990 (1982).
[9] PENG, I. C., und S. S. NIELSEN, J. Food Sci. **51**, 588—590 (1986).
[10] RIVAS, H. I., und P. SHERMAN, J. Dispersion Sci. Technol. **5**, 143 (1984).
[11] KURTH, L., Food Technol. Australia **35**, 420—423 (1983).
[12] KURTH, L., UND P. J. ROGERS, J. Food Sci. **49**, 573—576 (1984).
[13] MANN, E. J., Dairy Industries Intern. **50**, 11 (1985).
[14] MITTAL, G. S., und W. R. USBORNE, Food Technol. **39**, 121—130 (1985).
[15] BAWA, A. S., Functionality of fillers and extenders in meat emulsions. Diss. A., Univ. of Guelph, Guelph, Ontario, Canada 1984.
[16] HOLLAND, G. C., A meat industry perspective on the use of dairy ingredients, Proc. Conf. Canadian Dairy Ingredients in the Food Industry, Ottawa 1984.
[17] OELKER, P., unveröffentlichter Forschungsbericht, Zentralinstitut für Ernährung, Potsdam-Rehbrücke, 1985.
[18] COMER, F. W., N. CHEW, L. LOVELOCK und P. ALLAN-WOJTAS, Can. Inst. Food Sci. and Technol. **19**, 68—74 (1986).
[19] KATSARAS, S., und R. STENZEL, Fleischwirtsch. **64**, 955—957 (1984).
[20] RAEUBER, H.-J., I. KIESSLING und A. GEISSLER, Fleischwirtsch. **64**, 1375—1378 (1984).
[21] SIEGEL, D. G., K. E. CHURCH und G. R. SCHMIDT, J. Food Sci. **44**, 1276—1279 (1979).
[22] WALLINGFORD, L., und T.-P. LABUZA, J. Food Sci. **48**, 1—5 (1983).
[23] PUOLANNE, E., und M. RUUSUNEN, Fleischwirtsch. **63**, 631—633 (1983).

Dr. H. PETERS, Dr. J. KROLL und Prof. Dr. B. GASSMANN, Zentralinstitut für Ernährung, Arthur-Scheunert-Allee 114—116, Bergholz-Rehbrücke, DDR-1505

Eingegangen 10. 6. 1987

Die Nahrung 32 (1988) 9, 911—921

Zentralinstitut für Ernährung in Potsdam-Rehbrücke (Direktor: Prof. Dr. H. SCHMANDKE), Akademie der Wissenschaften der DDR, und Institut für Züchtungsforschung in Quedlinburg (Direktor: Prof. Dr. J. DEHNE), Akademie der Landwirtschaftswissenschaften der DDR

Zum Einfluß genetischer Merkmale und umweltspezifischer Faktoren auf die Zusammensetzung von Sojabohnen

G. MIETH, G. W. KRAUSSE, V. ERHARDT und K. MARZILGER

Es werden vergleichende Untersuchungen zur Zusammensetzung der Basiskomponenten und wertbestimmender Inhaltsstoffe von ausgewählten Sojabohnen-Sorten aus dem Weltsortiment (9 Genotypen) und von Dornburger-Neuzüchtungen (4 Mutationsstämme) durchgeführt. Dabei wird auch auf den Einfluß von Umweltfaktoren (3 Anbaugebiete, 9 Impfversuche) eingegangen. Die Ergebnisse werden unter ernährungsphysiologischen, anwendungstechnischen und züchterischen Aspekten diskutiert.

Einführung und Zielstellung

Sojabohnen spielen als Rohstoffquelle für hochwertige Nahrungsfette und Futterproteine seit längerem eine dominierende Rolle. Ihr Aufkommen im Weltmaßstab betrug 1985 beispielsweise 100,8 Mio t, das entspricht einem Gesamtpotential an Öl und Protein von ca. 20 bzw. 40 Mio. t [1].

Sieht man von den vielfältigen Verwertungsformen der Sojabohne als Grundnahrungsmittel im asiatischen Raum ab, so werden in anderen Regionen der Erde davon allerdings gegenwärtig nur insgesamt max. 2% — hauptsächlich in den USA — als Austausch — oder Zusatzstoffe für Lebensmittel direkt in der Humanernährung verwertet. Der Hauptanteil wird demgegenüber lediglich einer indirekten Veredlung über die Tierproduktion mit den bekannten Nachteilen hoher Transformationsverluste zugeführt [2].

Als Spitzenerzeuger für Sojabohnen fungieren derzeit die USA, Brasilien, China und Argentinien [1]. Seit dem letzten Dezennium wird auch dem Anbau spezieller, an die geographischen Gegebenheiten Mitteleuropas adaptierter Sorten, u. a. in der DDR, eine spezifische Bedeutung beigemessen [3]. Die Nutzbarmachung solcher neuen Sorten für eine Öl- und/oder Proteingewinnung setzt wiederum profunde Kenntnisse über ihre Zusammensetzung und die darauf einflußnehmenden genetischen, ökologischen, agrar- und verarbeitungstechnischen Faktoren voraus.

Es ist daher von Interesse, in der DDR kultivierte Genotypen (Standardsorten und Neuzuchtstämme) unterschiedlicher Provenienz hinsichtlich des Gehaltes wertbestimmender Inhaltsstoffe, speziell von Lipiden, Proteinen und antinutritiven Verbindungen, eingehender zu analysieren.

Material und Methoden

In das Untersuchungsprogramm wurden neben einigen Sorten der frühen und mittleren Reifegruppe des Weltsortiments als Vergleichssubstrate ausgewählte Dornburger Neuzüchtungen (GM) einbezogen (Tab. 1). Bei Stamm GM 1.55/82 erfolgte zum einen die Inhaltsstoffanalyse von neun Gliedern eines Impfversuches mit *Rhizobium japonicum*, wobei die Präparate jap. 1—6 aus dem FZB Müncheberg der AdL, der DDR, das Präparat jap. 7 aus der Versuchsstation Turda, SR Rumänien, stammte.

Zum anderen wurden Sojabohnen von nachstehend näher charakterisierten Standorten (Anbaujahr 1985) untersucht.

1. Dornburg (Bez. Gera)
   NStE: $Lö_1$ L/V AZ 62, ohne Düngung (Vorratsdüngung 1983), Vorfrucht Weizen
2. Beesenstedt (Bez. Halle)
   NStE: $Lö_1$ a AZ 71, Düngung: 40 kg N/ha, Impfung mit *Rhizobium jap.*,
   Vorfrucht Wintergerste

Tabelle 1
Angaben zum Genotyp und zur Herkunft der untersuchten Sojabohnen

Vers.-Block	Vers.-Nr.	Genotyp	Herkunftsland	Anbauort
I	1	Fiskeby V	Schweden	Dornburg
	2	Maple Arrow	Kanada	Dornburg
	3	Maple Presto	Kanada	Dornburg
	4	Gieso	BRD	Dornburg
	5	Niwa	UdSSR	Dornburg
	6	Niwa	UdSSR	Kiew
	7	Mc Call	USA	Dornburg
	8	KZ 761	Ungarn	Dornburg
	9	Dornburger Weißblühende	DDR	Dornburg
	10	GM. 1.53/82	DDR	Dornburg
	11	GM. 1.2088/82	DDR	Dornburg
	12	GM. 1.2128/82	DDR	Dornburg
	13	GM. 1.55/82	DDR	Dornburg
II	13	GM. 1.55/82	DDR	Dornburg
	14	GM. 1.55/82	DDR	Cobbelsdorf
	15	GM. 1.55/82	DDR	Beesenstedt
	16	GM. 1.55/82	DDR	Dornburg
		(ohne N., ohne Impf.)	DDR	Dornburg
	17	GM. 1.55/82 (40 kg N)	DDR	Dornburg
	18	GM. 1.55/82 (Impf. jap. 1)	DDR	Dornburg
	19	GM. 1.55/82 (Impf. jap. 2)	DDR	Dornburg
	20	GM. 1.55/82 (Impf. jap. 3)	DDR	Dornburg
	21	GM. 1.55/82 (Impf. jap. 4)	DDR	Dornburg
	22	GM. 1.55/82 (Impf. jap. 5)	DDR	Dornburg
	23	GM. 1.55/82 (Impf. jap. 6)	DDR	Dornburg
	24	GM. 1.55/82 (Impf. jap. 7)	DDR	Dornburg

3. Cobbelsdorf (Bez. Halle)
NStE: D2, 1S, AZ 26, ohne Düngung,
Vorfrucht Winterroggen.

Bezüglich der klimatischen Umwelteinflüsse ist folgendes anzumerken:

Die Sojabohnen gingen infolge optimaler Temperaturverhältnisse im Mai zum normalen Termin auf. Der relativ kühle Juni (2 °C unter langjährigem Mittel) führte zu einem um 2 Wochen verzögerten Blühbeginn und damit zu einer Verlangsamung der gesamten generativen Entwicklung. Ab Juli lagen die Monatstemperaturen im Bereich des langjährigen Mittels, die Niederschlagsmengen hingegen wesentlich darunter. Dadurch konnte die Reife der Sojabohnen ab September schnell voranschreiten und die frühe Reifegruppe noch Ende September/Anfang Oktober geerntet werden.

Die Bestimmung der Basiskomponenten von Sojabohnen erfolgte nach standardisierten Methoden der WEENDER-Futtermittelanalyse [4], die des Enzym-Inhibitor-Status spektrofotometrisch sowie die der Fett- und Aminosäurekomposition nach einschlägigen chromatographischen Arbeitsweisen [5].

Die statistischen Maßzahlen wurden in üblicher Weise berechnet. Der T-Test wurde nach COCHRAN (approximativer T-Test) durchgeführt, wobei im Versuchsblock I 13 verschiedenartige Genotypen, im Versuchsblock II der Stamm GM 1.55/82 von unterschiedlichen Standorten, einschließlich einer Düngung und Beimpfung, zusammengefaßt wurde.

Ergebnisse und Diskussion

Angaben zum Gehalt der für eine Weiterverarbeitung der Sojabohnen besonders interessierenden Sameninhaltsstoffe ausgewählter Genotypen und Herkünfte sind in den

Tabelle 2
Basiskomponenten verschiedenartiger Sojabohnen-Genotypen und -Provenienz

Versuchs-Nr.	Rohprotein [%]	Reinfett [%]	Rohfaser [%]	N-freie Extraktstoffe [%]	Wasser [%]	Schalen [%]	TKM [g]
1	33,1	15,3	4,6	29,3	7,0	7,7	147,8
2	36,7	16,1	4,7	22,1	8,9	8,2	165,0
3	36,9	15,3	4,3	22,4	7,4	6,7	131,7
4	33,9	13,0	4,6	27,1	7,2	7,7	144,0
5	38,3	14,1	4,5	20,0	7,9	7,3	126,3
6	36,5	15,2	4,4	22,9	7,8	7,2	139,7
7	34,2	14,6	4,2	26,0	7,6	6,5	150,3
8	35,6	13,4	4,5	25,4	6,7	7,4	146,3
9	40,7	12,9	5,2	26,9	6,9	9,2	94,8
10	29,0	15,3	4,6	28,5	6,3	7,6	144,2
11	35,0	13,4	4,8	24,2	6,9	8,2	148,0
12	34,5	15,2	4,4	28,3	6,7	7,0	163,7
13	35,1	14,0	5,0	22,8	7,2	8,6	135,5
14	29,0	16,7	4,9	24,6	11,4	8,4	149,3
15	42,2	14,2	5,1	19,2	11,8	9,1	152,2
16	31,6	14,8	4,7	26,8	6,6	8,0	134,8
17	32,1	15,3	5,1	25,7	6,1	8,9	138,6
18	31,1	15,6	5,0	25,5	6,3	8,6	133,2
19	35,5	13,8	4,8	24,0	6,7	8,3	127,3
20	34,4	14,3	5,1	24,1	5,9	9,1	132,7
21	35,8	14,8	4,6	21,4	6,5	7,5	130,2
22	34,7	14,2	5,2	29,0	6,5	9,2	130,6
23	34,9	14,6	4,6	21,2	6,7	7,7	129,8
24	35,2	13,9	5,0	24,5	6,5	8,6	134,0

Tab. 2—6 zusammengestellt. Die zugehörigen statistischen Maßzahlen und Korrelationen finden sich in den Tab. 6 und 7. Die erhaltenen Ergebnisse sind wie folgt zu interpretieren:

Verschiedenartige Sojabohnen weisen erwartungsgemäß mehr oder weniger gravierende Unterschiede in ihrer Zusammensetzung auf, die auf genetische Merkmale und umweltspezifische Einflüsse zurückzuführen sind. So belaufen sich bei 9 Genotypen aus dem internationalen Standardsortiment und 4 Mutationsstämmen aus dem Dornburger Neuzuchtprogramm die Rohproteingehalte auf 29,0 bis 42,2% ($\bar{x}$ 34,8%), die Reinfettgehalte auf 12,9 bis 16,1% ($\bar{x}$ 14,4%), die Rohfasergehalte auf 4,2 bis 5,2% ($\bar{x}$ 4,6%), die Gehalte an stickstofffreien Extraktstoffen auf 20,0 bis 29,3% ($\bar{x}$ 25,1%) und die Schalengehalte auf 6,7 bis 9,2% ($\bar{x}$ 7,6%). Erhebliche, insbesondere genotypische Unterschiede bestehen im weiteren zwischen der Tausend-Korn-Masse, die zwischen 94,8 und 165,0 g ($\bar{x}$ 141,3 g) schwankt. Der höchste Rohproteingehalt entfällt dabei mit 43,7% i. T. auf die mittelspäte Sorte „Dornburger Weißblühende", der höchste Reinfettgehalt mit 17,7% i. T. auf die kanadische Sorte „Maple Arrow" (Tab. 2).

Der Einfluß der Umweltfaktoren zeigt sich deutlich am Beispiel des Zuchtstammes 1.55/82, der in Abhängigkeit von Standort, Düngung und Beimpfung eine Variabilität im Rohproteingehalt von 29,0 bis 42,2% ($\bar{x}$ 34,3%), im Reinfettgehalt von 13,8 bis 16,7% ($\bar{x}$ 14,7%), im Rohfasergehalt von 4,6 bis 5,1% ($\bar{x}$ 4,9%), im Gehalt an stickstofffreien

Tabelle 3
Enzym- und Inhibitor-Aktivitäten verschiedenartiger Sojabohnen-Genotypen und -Provenienz

Versuchs-Nr.	Lipoxygenase-Aktivität [g^{-1} min^{-1}]	Urease-Aktivität [ΔpH]	Trypsininhibitor-Aktivität [mg/g]
1	75,0	2,13	27,0
2	101,6	2,10	27,8
3	75,3	2,11	26,8
4	75,5	2,17	25,1
5	61,5	2,11	24,3
6	44,3	2,17	29,3
7	60,1	2,07	23,3
8	86,6	2,06	27,5
9	68,6	2,02	21,1
10	70,5	2,14	31,2
11	75,0	2,03	27,2
12	75,9	2,09	23,5
13	76,3	2,10	28,5
14	72,5	2,12	32,0
15	74,3	2,06	31,8
16	76,6	2,09	32,4
17	61,7	2,12	33,5
18	60,6	2,14	33,3
19	70,1	2,12	34,2
20	62.1	2,00	31,8
21	62,5	2,06	33,9
22	97,0	2,09	30,0
23	70,0	2,12	32,0
24	55,4	2,05	32,6

Extraktstoffen von 19,2 bis 29,0% ($\bar{x}$ 24,1%), im Schalengehalt von 7,5 bis 9,1% ($\bar{x}$ 8,5%) und in der Tausend-Korn-Masse von 127,3 bis 152,2 g ($\bar{x}$ 135,7 g) aufweist. Dabei ist der Standorteinfluß besonders markant, wogegen Stickstoffdüngung und Beimpfung mit *Rhizobium jap.* geringere Auswirkungen zeigen (Tab. 2).

Im Enzym- und Enzym-Inhibitor-Status sind zwischen den Genotypen und Herkünften gleichfalls spezifische Unterschiede charakteristisch. Diese betreffen vor allem die Lipoxygenase-Aktivität mit einer Variabilität von 44,3 bis 101,6 g^{-1} min^{-1} ($\bar{x}$ 71,9 g^{-1} min^{-1}), wie auch die Trypsin-Inhibitor-Aktivität mit einer solchen zwischen 21,1 und 34,2 mg/g ($\bar{x}$ 29,1 mg/g), wogegen sich die Urease-Aktivität mit Werten von 2,00 bis 2,17 ΔpH ($\bar{x}$ 2,1 Δ pH) geringfügiger voneinander unterscheidet. Im Fall von Lipoxygenase ist dabei auf einen erheblichen Einfluß von Sorte und Stickstoffdüngung, bei Trypsin-Inhibitoren auf einen solchen von Sorte und Standort hinzuweisen (Tab. 3).

Die genetische und durch Umweltfaktoren bedingte Varianz des Fettsäurespektrums von Sojabohnen ist unter den ausgewählten Standort- und Anbaubedingungen relativ gering. So belaufen sich bei allen Versuchsmustern die Schwankungen im relativen Gehalt an Palmitinsäure auf 8,9 bis 13,3% ($\bar{x}$ 11,5%), Stearinsäure auf 3,1 bis 4,5% ($\bar{x}$ 3,6%), Ölsäure auf 14,2 bis 19,2% ($\bar{x}$ 16,3%), Linolsäure auf 53,6 bis 57,1% ($\bar{x}$ 54,9%) und Linolensäure auf 11,1 bis 15,4% ($\bar{x}$ 13,2%). Auffällig sind die hohen Gehalte an Linolensäure und ein

Tabelle 4
Fettsäuren-Zusammensetzung verschiedenartiger Sojabohnen-Genotypen und -Provenienz

Versuchs-Nr.	Palmitinsäure		Stearinsäure		Ölsäure		Linolsäure		Linolensäure	
	[%]	[% rel.]	[%]	[% rel.]	[%]	[% rel.]	[%]	[% rel.]	[%]	[% rel.]
1	1,8	11,8	0,5	3,2	2,5	16,6	8,5	55,8	1,9	12,6
2	1,6	10,0	0,5	3,2	2,7	17,1	9,0	56,0	2,2	13,6
3	1,5	10,0	0,5	3,4	2,8	18,2	8,3	54,8	2,1	13,6
4	1,7	13,3	0,5	3,9	2,4	18,5	6,8	53,6	1,5	11,8
5	1,5	9,7	0,6	4,0	3,4	19,2	8,0	53,0	1,7	11,1
6	1,4	10,2	0,5	3,7	2,4	16,8	7,8	55,1	2,0	14,2
7	1,4	9,5	0,5	3,5	2,5	17,3	8,4	54,5	1,8	12,3
8	1,2	9,2	0,7	4,5	2,3	17,2	7,5	55,7	2,0	14,6
9	1,3	10,3	0,5	3,6	2,0	15,5	6,9	54,3	2,1	15,4
10	2,0	13,4	0,6	3,8	2,6	16,1	8,3	54,3	1,8	11,8
11	1,7	12,4	0,5	3,8	2,1	15,7	7,3	54,6	1,8	13,6
12	1,8	12,1	0,5	3,4	2,3	15,1	8,4	55,5	2,1	14,0
13	1,7	11,9	0,5	3,2	2,0	14,2	7,9	56,3	2,0	14,4
14	2,1	12,4	0,6	3,6	2,7	16,2	9,3	55,4	2,1	12,4
15	1,8	12,9	0,6	4,1	2,5	17,7	7,7	54,2	1,6	11,2
16	1,9	12,8	0,5	3,1	2,4	15,9	8,2	55,7	1,8	12,5
17	1,9	12,4	0,6	3,7	2,4	15,8	8,5	55,2	2,0	12,9
18	2,1	13,2	0,6	3,6	2,5	16,2	8,5	54,7	1,9	12,3
19	1,7	12,2	0,5	3,8	2,1	15,5	7,6	55,2	1,8	13,3
20	1,8	12,6	0,5	3,3	2,2	15,4	7,9	54,9	2,0	14,0
21	1,8	12,0	0,5	3,5	2,3	15,5	8,1	54,4	2,2	14,6
22	1,3	8,9	0,5	3,5	2,3	16,3	7,7	54,2	2,0	13,8
23	1,8	12,0	0,5	3,6	2,2	15,1	8,0	55.1	2.1	14,2
24	1,6	11,3	0,5	3,7	2,0	14,7	7,9	57.1	1,8	13,2

rel. = bezogen auf den Fettgehalt der Bohnen

dazu korrespondierendes hohes Verteilungsverhältnis von ungesättigten zu gesättigten Fettsäuren (Tab. 4).

In der Aminosäurekomposition, speziell dem Anteil der essentiellen Aminosäuren Lysin, Methionin und Cystein, sind gravierende Effekte von genetischen Merkmalen und Umwelteinflüssen gleichfalls nicht erkennbar. Dabei ist jedoch zu berücksichtigen, daß die Auswirkungen einer unterschiedlichen Stickstoffversorgung im Rahmen der Versuchsserie aus technischen Gründen nicht erfaßt werden konnten. Die Schwankungsbreite der relativen Gehalte beträgt für Lysin 5,5 bis 6,7 g/16 g N ($\bar{x}$ 6,1 g/16 g N), Methionin 1,2 bis 1,8 g/16 g N ($\bar{x}$ 1,5 g/16 g N) und Cystein 1,3 bis 2,1 g/16 g N ($\bar{x}$ 1,6 g/16 g N) (Tab. 5).

Statistisch signifikante Differenzen in der Zusammensetzung der in den beiden Versuchsblöcken zusammengefaßten Genotypen und Herkünfte bestehen lediglich bezüglich des Rohfaser- und Schalengehaltes, der Trypsin-Inhibitor-Aktivität sowie des Anteils an Palmitinsäure und Cystein (Tab. 6). Die untersuchten Genotypen unterscheiden sich somit in der Zusammensetzung ihrer Basiskomponenten und im Gehalt anderer wertbestimmender Inhaltsstoffe nur unwesentlich von den Herkünften. In Übereinstimmung mit Ergebnissen anderer Arbeitsgruppen wirken sich somit bei Sojabohnen sortenspezifische Unterschiede in der Regel weniger gravierend auf die Zusammensetzung aus als Umweltbedingungen. Diese betreffen insbesondere die markanten Einflüsse klimatischer Faktoren auf den Fett- und Proteingehalt sowie das Spektrum der Fett- und Aminosäuren [6—9].

Was Zusammenhänge zwischen den einzelnen Prüfgrößen angeht, so ist für den Rohproteingehalt einerseits eine negative Korrelation zum Gehalt an Reinfett, stickstofffreien Extraktstoffen, der Urease-Aktivität und der Tausend-Korn-Masse, andererseits eine positive Korrelation zum Gehalt an Schalen, Lysin, Methionin und Cystein charakteristisch.

Tabelle 5
Aminosäuren-Zusammensetzung verschiedenartiger Sojabohnen-Genotypen und -Provenienz

Aminosäure [g/16 g N]	Versuchs-Nr.						
	1	2	3	4	5	6	7
Asparaginsäure	3,7 (11,1)	4,3 (11,6)	4,2 (11,3)	3,9 (11,7)	4,2 (10,9)	3,9 (10,1)	4,0 (11,6)
Threonin	1,3 (3,9)	1,4 (3,8)	1,4 (3,8)	1,3 (3,9)	1,4 (3,6)	1,3 (3,4)	1,4 (4,1)
Serin	1,4 (4,2)	1,6 (4,3)	1,6 (4,3)	1,4 (4,2)	1,5 (3,9)	1,4 (3,6)	1,5 (4,4)
Glutaminsäure	5,6 (16,8)	6,2 (16,7)	6,2 (16,7)	5,7 (17,1)	6,9 (17,9)	6,0 (15,6)	6,2 (18,0)
Prolin	1,8 (5,4)	1,8 (4,9)	2,0 (5,4)	1,9 (5,7)	2,2 (5,7)	2,0 (5,2)	2,0 (5,8)
Cystin/2	0,5 (1,5)	0,6 (1,6)	0,6 (1,6)	0,5 (1,5)	0,5 (1,3)	0,6 (1,6)	0,5 (1,5)
Glycin	1,5 (4,5)	1,6 (4,3)	1,6 (4,3)	1,5 (4,5)	1,6 (4,2)	1,5 (3,9)	1,6 (4,6)
Valin	1,6 (4,8)	1,7 (5,0)	1,7 (5,0)	1,7 (5,1)	1,9 (4,9)	1,7 (4,4)	1,8 (5,2)
Alanin	1,4 (4,2)	1,5 (4,1)	1,5 (4,1)	1,5 (4,5)	1,6 (4,2)	1,6 (4,2)	1,5 (4,4)
Methionin	0,5 (1,5)	0,6 (1,6)	0,6 (1,6)	0,5 (1,5)	0,6 (1,6)	0,6 (1,6)	0,4 (1,2)
Isoleucin	1,6 (4,8)	1,7 (5,0)	1,6 (4,3)	1,6 (4,8)	1,7 (4,4)	1,6 (4,2)	1,7 (4,9)
Leucin	2,4 (7,2)	2,6 (7,0)	2,6 (7,0)	2,5 (7,5)	2,7 (7,0)	2,5 (6,5)	2,6 (7,5)
Tyrosin	1,1 (3,3)	1,2 (3,2)	1,2 (3,2)	1,1 (3,3)	1,3 (3,4)	1,1 (2,9)	1,1 (3,2)
Phenylalanin	1,8 (5,4)	1,9 (5,1)	1,9 (5,1)	1,6 (4,8)	2,0 (5,2)	1,8 (4,7)	1,7 (4,9)
Histidin	1,0 (3,0)	1,1 (3,0)	1,1 (3,0)	1,0 (3,0)	1,1 (2,9)	1,0 (2,6)	1,0 (2,9)
Ornithin	0,03 (0,1)	0,04 (0,1)	0,03 (0,1)	0,04 (0,1)	0,04 (0,1)	0,06 (0,2)	0,04 (0,1)
Lysin	2,1 (6,3)	2,2 (5,9)	2,2 (5,9)	2,0 (6,0)	2,3 (6,0)	2,1 (5,5)	2,2 (6,4)
Arginin	2,2 (6,6)	2,4 (6,5)	2,4 (6,5)	2,2 (6,6)	2,6 (6,8)	2,4 (6,2)	2,7 (7,8)

Weitere Korrelationen betreffen die Fett- und Aminosäurekomposition und zwar dahingehend, daß mit steigendem Fettgehalt der Anteil essentieller Linol- und Linolensäure, mit steigendem Proteingehalt jedoch der Anteil an essentiellem Lysin, Methionin und Cystein zunimmt (Tab. 7). Letzteres steht im Widerspruch zu bekannten tendenziellen Zusammenhängen, wonach bei Sojabohnen zwischen der Quantität und Qualität von Lipiden und Proteinen im allgemeinen eine umgekehrte Proportionalität besteht. Die gleichermaßen niedrigen Fett- und Proteingehalte weisen jedoch auf Überlagerungseffekte verschiedenartiger ungünstiger Umweltfaktoren (geographische Lage, Klima, Nährstoffversorgung, Fotoperiode) hin, da normalerweise bei kälteren Standorten u. a. die Proteinsynthese zu Lasten der Fettsynthese stimuliert wird [10—14]. Hierzu ist jedoch einschränkend festzustellen, daß die relativ geringe Anzahl der Versuchsdaten nur eine begrenzte Verallgemeinerung zuläßt.

Aus ernährungsphysiologischer Sicht ist der hohe Gehalt an essentiellen Fettsäuren günstig zu beurteilen, wenn auch ein hoher Anteil von Linolensäure verarbeitungstechnische Probleme bedingt. Als günstig im Hinblick auf den Futterwert von entfetteten Sojabohnen ist auch der hohe Gehalt an essentiellen Eckaminosäuren zu beurteilen. Dabei ist jedoch zu berücksichtigen, daß die genetische Variabilität der Fettsäure- wie auch der Aminosäurekomposition von Sojabohnen relativ gering ist und maßgeblich durch Umwelteinflüsse geprägt wird [10—14].

Aus anwendungsorientierter Sicht einer Verwertung von Sojabohnen in der Tier- und/oder Humanernährung sind die auffälligen beidermaßen niedrigen Fett- und Proteingehalte der auf DDR-Standorten kultivierten Sojabohnen ökonomisch wenig attraktiv. Eine

Versuchs-Nr.							
8	9	10	11	12	13	14	15
4,3 (12,0)	4,3 (10,8)	3,3 (11,6)	3,8 (11,0)	3,7 (10,7)	3,7 (10,7)	3,5 (12,3)	4,4 (10,6)
1,5 (4,2)	1,5 (3,8)	1,2 (4,2)	1,3 (3,8)	1,3 (3,8)	1,3 (3,8)	1,2 (4,2)	1,4 (3,4)
1,6 (4,5)	1,7 (4,3)	1,3 (4,6)	1,5 (4,4)	1,4 (4,1)	1,4 (4,1)	1,3 (4,6)	1,6 (3,8)
6,3 (17,6)	6,8 (17,0	4,8 (16,8)	5,7 (16,5)	5,7 (16,5)	5,7 (16,5)	5,2 (18,2)	7,0 (16,8)
2,0 (5,6)	2,2 (5,5)	1,6 (5,6)	2,0 (5,8)	1,8 (5,2)	1,8 (5,2)	1,7 (6,0)	2,2 (5,3)
0,5 (1,4)	0,6 (1,5)	0,5 (1,8)	0,5 (1,5)	0,5 (1,5)	0,6 (1,7)	0,6 (2,1)	0,6 (1,4)
1,6 (4,5)	1,7 (4,3)	1,3 (4,6)	1,4 (4,1)	1,5 (4,4)	1,5 (4,4)	1,4 (4,9)	1,7 (4,2)
1,8 (5,0)	1,9 (4,8)	1,5 (5,3)	1,6 (4,6)	1,7 (4,9)	1,6 (4,6)	1,5 (5,3)	1,9 (4,6)
1,6 (4,5)	1,6 (4,0)	1,3 (4,6)	1,4 (4,1)	1,4 (4,1)	1,4 (4,1)	1,3 (4,6)	1,6 (3,8)
0,5 (1,4)	0,6 (1,5)	0,5 (1,8)	0,6 (1,7)	0,5 (1,5)	0,5 (1,5)	0,5 (1,8)	0,6 (1,4)
1,7 (4,8)	1,8 (4,5)	1,4 (4,9)	1,6 (4,6)	1,5 (4,4)	1,6 (4,6)	1,4 (4,9)	1,8 (4,3)
2,7 (7,6)	2,8 (7,0)	2,1 (7,4)	2,4 (7,0)	2,4 (7,0)	2,4 (7,0)	2,2 (7,7)	2,8 (6,7)
1,2 (3,4)	1,3 (3,3)	1,0 (3,5)	1,1 (3,2)	1,1 (3,2)	1,2 (3,5)	1,0 (3,5)	1,3 (3,1)
1,9 (5,3)	2,0 (5,0)	1,5 (5,3)	1,7 (4,9)	1,8 (5,2)	1,8 (5,2)	1,6 (5,6)	2,1 (5,0)
1,1 (3,1)	1,1 (2,8)	0,8 (2,8)	1,0 (2,9)	1,1 (3,2)	1,0 (2,9)	0,9 (3,2)	1,1 (2,6)
0,03 (0,1)	0,03 (0,1)	0,02 (0,1)	0,06 (0,2)	0,04 (0,1)	0,03 (0,1)	0,03 (0,1)	0,04 (0,1)
2,2 (6,2)	2,3 (5,8)	1,9 (6,7)	2,2 (6,4)	2,2 (6,4)	2,3 (6,7)	1,9 (6,7)	2,5 (6,0)
2,4 (6,7)	2,9 (7,3)	1,8 (6,3)	2,4 (7,0)	2,6 (7,5)	2,5 (7,3)	2,0 (7,0)	3,0 (7,2)

Tabelle 6
Statistische Maßzahlen zu den Tabellen 2 bis 5

Tab. Nr.	Inhaltsstoff	Mittelwert			Stand. Abweichung			Stand. Fehler			Signifik.
		gesamt	Block 1	Block 2	gesamt	Block 1	Block 2	gesamt	Block 1	Block 2	T-Test
2	Rohprotein	34,8	35,3	34,3	3,1	2,8	3,3	0,6	0,8	0,9	0,599
	Reinfett	14,6	14,4	14,7	1,0	1,0	0,8	0,2	0,3	0,2	0,463
	Rohfaser	4,7	4,6	4,9	0,3	0,3	0,2	0,06	0,08	0,06	0,997
	N-fr. Extrakt	24,7	25,1	24,1	2,8	2,9	2,7	0,6	0,8	0,8	0,624
	Wasser	7,3	7,3	7,4	1,5	0,7	2,0	0,3	0,2	0,6	0,103
	Schalen	8,0	7,6	8,5	0,8	0,8	0,6	0,2	0,2	0,2	0,996
	TKM	138,8	141,3	135,7	14,2	17,8	7,7	2,9	4,9	2,2	0,690
3	Lipoxyg.-Akt.	71,2	73,1	69,9	12,4	14,1	11,0	2,5	4,1	3,2	0,461
	Urease-Akt.	2,1	2,1	2,1	0,04	0,05	0,04	0,1	0,01	0,01	0,433
	Trypsininh.-Akt.	29,1	26,4	32,2	3,8	2,8	1,6	0,8	0,8	0,5	1,00
4	Palmitinsäure	1,7	1,6	1,8	0,2	0,2	0,2	0,05	0,06	0,06	0,972
	Stearinsäure	0,5	0,5	0,5	0,06	0,06	0,05	0,01	0,02	0,01	0,090
	Ölsäure	2,4	2,5	2,3	0,3	0,4	0,2	0,06	0,1	0,06	0,803
	Linolsäure	8,0	7,9	8,1	0,6	0,7	0,5	0,1	0,2	0,1	0,557
	Linolensäure	1,9	1,9	1,9	0,2	0,2	0,2	0,04	0,05	0,05	0,199
5	Asparaginsäure	3,9	3,9	3,8	0,3	0,3	0,4	0,09	0,09	0,3	0,193
	Threonin	1,3	1,4	1,3	0,09	0,09	0,1	0,02	0,02	0,06	0,547
	Serin	1,5	1,5	1,4	0,1	0,1	0,2	0,03	0,03	0,09	0,378
	Glutaminsäure	6,0	6,0	6,0	0,6	0,5	0,9	0,2	0,2	0,5	0,023
	Prolin	1,9	1,9	1,9	0,2	0,2	0,3	0,05	0,05	0,2	0,135
	Cystin/2	0,5	0,5	0,6	0,05	0,05	0,0	0,01	0,01	0,0	0,999
	Glycin	1,5	1,5	1,5	0,1	0,1	0,2	0,03	0,03	0,09	0,020
	Alanin	1,5	1,5	1,4	0,1	0,1	0,2	0,03	0,03	0,09	0,366
	Valin	1,7	1,7	1,7	0,1	0,1	0,2	0,03	0,03	0,1	0,227
	Methionin	0,5	0,5	0,5	0,06	0,07	0,06	0,02	0,02	0,03	0,099
	Isoleucin	1,6	1,6	1,6	0,1	0,1	0,2	0,03	0,03	0,1	0,136
	Leucin	2,5	2,5	2,5	0,2	0,2	0,3	0,05	0,05	0,2	0,185
	Tyrosin	1,2	1,2	1,2	0,1	0,09	0,2	0,03	0,02	0,09	0,099
	Phenylalanin	1,8	1,8	1,8	0,2	0,1	0,3	0,04	0,04	0,1	0,154

Histidin	1,0	1,0	1,0	0,09	0,09	0,1	0,02	0,02	0,06	0,344
Ornithin	0,04	0,04	0,03	0,01	0,01	0,006	0,003	0,003	0,03	0,621
Lysin	2,2	2,2	2,2	0,2	0,1	0,3	0,04	0,03	0,2	0,245
Arginin	2,4	2,4	2,2	0,3	0,3	0,8	0,08	0,07	0,4	0,376

Tabelle 7
Korrelationen zwischen ausgewählten Inhaltsstoffen von Sojabohnen

Rohprotein	Reinfett	N-fr. Extrakt	Schalen	Lysin	Methionin	Cystin/2
normal	−0,4986(+)	−0,5390(++)	0,4525(+)	0,8934 (+++)	0,6245(++)	—
SPEARMAN Rank	−0,4099(+)	−0,6380(+++)	—	0,81689(+++)	0,7753(++)	0,4798(+)
Reinfett	**Urease-Akt.**	**Linolsäure**	**Linolensäure**	**TKM**		
normal	0,4092(+)	0,9403(+++)	0,4443(+)	0,4525(+)		
SPEARMAN Rank	0,4609(+)	0,9112(+++)	0,4007(+)	—		
Cystin/2	**Methionin**	**Lysin**				
normal	0,4812(+)	—				
SPEARMAN Rank	0,4841(+)	0,4272(+)				

Die Angaben für Fett- und Aminosäuren beziehen sich auf %

nähere Betrachtung der drei Herkünfte des Neuzuchtstammes GM 1.55/82 führt jedoch zu der Schlußfolgerung, daß eine kombinierte Stickstoffdüngung und Beimpfung mit *Rhizobium jap.* (Standort Beesenstedt) eine deutliche Anhebung des Proteingehaltes bis auf 42,3 % bedingt, wogegen auf den beiden anderen, schlechter mit Stickstoff versorgten Standorten nur Rohproteingehalte zwischen 29 und 35 % nachgewiesen wurden. In Übereinstimmung damit wird auch in den meisten Impfversuchen ein höherer Rohproteingehalt erzielt, während eine alleinige Düngung mit 40 kg N/ha sich nur geringfügig darauf auswirkt.

Unter züchterischen Aspekten ist zum einen die negative Korrelation zwischen dem Rohprotein- und Fettgehalt sowie zwischen Rohproteingehalt und Tausendkornmasse, zum anderen aber eine hohe Kornertragsleistung auch unter kühleren Klimabedingungen von besonderem Interesse. Für Produktionsbelange ist ein hoher Rohproteinertrag bei akzeptablem Fettgehalt, früher Kornreife und Mähdruscheignung wesentlich. Diesen vielseitigen Ansprüchen dürfte der Zuchtstamm GM 1.55/82, der durch Mutationsauslösung aus der schwedischen Sorte „Fiskeby V" hervorgegangen ist und sich in der Zusammensetzung seiner Inhaltsstoffe nur wenig von dieser unterscheidet, am ehesten entsprechen.

Summary

G. MIETH, K. W. KRAUSSE, V. ERHARDT and K. MARZILGER: Influence of genetic and environmental factors on the composition of soybeans

The composition of value-determining basic and minor components of soybeans of 9 genotypes selected from the world collection and of 4 mutation lines from the national breeding programme of the GDR are determined. In this connection the influence of the environment is taken into consideration, too. The results are discussed according to the nutritive value and the cultivation project as well as to application field of soybean products for human nutrition and animal feeding.

Резюме

Г. МИТ, Г. В. КРАУСЕ, В. ЭРХАРДТ и К. МАРЦИЛГЕР: Влияние генетических показателей и специфических факторов окружающей среды на состав соевых бобов

Проводились сравнительные исследования состава основных компонентов и определяющих ценность составных веществ избранных сортов соевых бобов из мирового ассортимента (9 генотипов) и Дорнбургских новых селективных сортов (4 мутации). При этом обратили внимание и на влияние факторов окружающей среды (3 места выращивания, 9 опытов прививки). Результаты обсуждаются с точки зрения физиологии питания, технологии использования и селекции.

Literatur

[1] FAO Production Yearbook 1984, Rome 1985.
[2] SCHWENKE, K. D., Eiweißquellen der Zukunft, Urania-Verlag, Leipzig, Jena, Berlin 1985.
[3] KRAUSSE, G. W., R. ALBRECHT, M. ZACCHARIAS und H. E. SCHMIDT, Eurosoya **4**, 99 (1986).
[4] Fachbereichsstandards (TGL) der Land-, Forst- und Nahrungsgüterwirtschaft, Berlin 1985.
[5] Methodenkatalog des ZfE der AdW, Bergholz-Rehbrücke 1985.

[6] Marquard, R. A., Einfluß von Standortfaktoren und spezifischen Klimakonstellationen auf Fettgehalt, Fettsäurezusammensetzung und Tokopherolgehalt von Raps, Sonnenblumen, Soja und Lein, Habilitationsschrift, Justus-Liebig-Univ., Gießen 1980.
[7] Schuster, W., Fett/Wissenschaft Technologie **89**, 15 (1987).
[8] Makusko, J. P., und V. F. Baranov, Soja, Kolos-Verlag, Moskau 1984.
[9] Schütt, Weltwirtschaftspflanzen, Verlag Paul Parey, Berlin und Hamburg 1972.
[10] Martin, B. A., R. R. Wilson und R. W. Rinne, J. am. Oil Chem. Soc. **63**, 346 (1986).
[11] Cherry, J. H., Food Sci. Technol. Abstr. **17**/11, 140 (1985).
[12] Zlamal, P., und V. Marek, Genetika a Slechteni **17**, 89 (1981).
[13] Karlubik, M., Z. Dusan und D. Dusan, Polnohospodarstvo **26**, 722 (1980).
[14] Carls, J., Acker- und Pflanzenbau **153**, 274 (1984).

Dr. G. Mieth, Dr. V. Erhardt und Karin Marzilger, Zentralinstitut für Ernährung, Arthur-Scheunert-Allee 114—116, Bergholz-Rehbrücke, DDR-1505, und Prof. Dr. G. W. Krausse, Institut für Züchtungsforschung, Postfach 225, Quedlinburg, DDR-4300

Eingegangen 10. 6. 1987

Die Nahrung 32 (1988) 9, 922—923

Rezensionen

J. Straus: **Gewerblicher Rechtsschutz für biotechnologische Erfindungen.** 86 Seiten. Carl Heymanns Verlag KG, Köln u. a. 1987. Preis: 40,— DM.

Der Autor hat die vorliegende Schrift, bei der es sich um eine Studie zur Analyse einiger Grundsatzfragen zu biotechnologischen Erfindungen handelt, auf Ersuchen des Internationalen Büros der Weltorganisation für geistiges Eigentum (WIPO) in Genf erstellt. Einige Probleme, die in den letzten Jahrzehnten eine zunehmende Bedeutung für die Ausdehnung des Patentrechtes auf biotechnologische Erfindungen erlangt haben, werden besonders behandelt. Dazu gehören:

— was stellt eine biotechnologische Erfindung dar,
— welche technologischen Entwicklungen sind auf diesem Gebiet zu berücksichtigen,
— sind bestimmte biotechnologische Erfindungen von einem Patentschutz auszuschließen,
— welche Patentierungsvoraussetzungen sind auf biotechnologische Erfindungen anzuwenden?

Die Studie geht in gestraffter Form und übersichtlicher Weise zunächst auf Merkmale zur Einführung eindeutiger Begriffe der Biotechnologie ein und behandelt unter Anwendung solcher Begriffe traditionelle Methoden der Züchtung von Pflanzen und Tieren sowie den Einsatz von Mikroorganismen. Daran anschließend werden die neuen Technologien und Kategorien biotechnologischer Erfindungen abgehandelt.

In einem weiteren Abschnitt wird auf den gewerblichen Rechtsschutz für biotechnologische Erfindungen auf nationaler Ebene eingegangen. Dabei wird sowohl der Schutz von Pflanzensorten und Tierarten, als auch insbesondere die Anwendung der Patentierungsvoraussetzungen auf biotechnologische Erfindungen berücksichtigt. Die Studie gewinnt eine besondere Bedeutung durch zahlreiche in ihr berücksichtigte und angeführte Literaturstellen. Die Schrift des als Experte geschätzten Autors dürfte besonderes Interesse finden bei Patentrechtlern, die mit der Entwicklung und Weiterentwicklung des gewerblichen Rechtsschutzes für biotechnologische Erfindungen befaßt sind, aber auch bei Biotechnologen, die sich mit diesem speziellen Fachgebiet und den Entwicklungstendenzen bekannt machen wollen. Rinck

Handbuch apparativer Verfahren in der Psychologie. Herausgegeben von R. Brickenkamp. 562 Seiten, zahlr. Abb. und Tab. Verlag für Psychologie, Dr. C. J. Hogrefe, Göttingen, Toronto, Zürich 1986. Preis: 198,— DM.

Aus den mehr als 100 Jahren experimenteller psychologischer Forschung existiert ein fast unübersehbarer Bestand technischer Hilfsmittel und Apparate, der im vorliegenden Handbuch klassifiziert und mit methodischer und technischer Detailinformation vorgestellt wird. Behandelt werden sowohl die ersten experimentellen Versuchsanordnungen von Weber und Fechner im 19. Jahrhundert und mechanische und elektromechanische Eigenbauten, die bis in die 50er Jahre unseres Jahrhunderts dauerten, als auch hochentwickelte, elektronische Geräte, die als Folge der sogenannten „zweiten industriellen Revolution" im psychologischen Apparatebestand in den 60er Jahren bis 1986 auf den Markt kamen. Gebräuchliche apparative Verfahren wichtiger Funktionsprinzipien werden allgemeinverständlich mit Hinweisen auf die Einsatzgebiete und die Anwendungsmöglichkeiten dargestellt: einfache Zeitmeßgeräte, Ton- und Bildaufzeichnungs- und Wiedergabegeräte, apparative Verfahren zur Prüfung der grundlegenden Funktionen der visuellen und akustischen Wahrnehmung, Geräte zur Messung der Flimmerverschmelzungsfrequenz, Tachistoskope, Apparate zur Messung von Aufmerksamkeit, Konzentration und Vigilanz sowie Reaktionszeitmeßgeräte ferner Determinationsgeräte zur Untersuchung des Verhaltens bei psychophysischer Belastung (Streß, Alkohol, Drogen), apparative Prüfverfahren psychomotorischer Fertigkeiten und Apparaturen für die experimentelle Lernpsychologie. Psychophysiologische Meßverfahren und -apparaturen stellen mit über 100 Seiten einen Schwerpunkt dar. Sie erlauben die Messung physiologischer Veränderungen und Prozesse, die für psychologische Vorgänge wie Trieb, Motivation, Haltung, Gefühl von Bedeutung sind. Die Textbeiträge sind allgemein verständlich, bieten Bewertungen und z. T. Hinweise für wünschenswerte Weiterentwicklungen. Sie werden durch Fotografien, Schemata, Literaturhinweise und tabellarische Einzeldarstellungen ergänzt. Vier nachgestellte Register ermöglichen eine leichte Orientierung: Namen- und Sachregister, alphabetisches Verzeichnis von über 400 Geräten einschließlich Hersteller sowie Anschriftenverzeichnis der Hersteller und Vertriebsfirmen.

G. Lewerenz

E. SATTER: **How to get your kid to eat — but not too much.** 396Seiten. Bull Publishing Co., Palo Alto, CA, 1987.

Die wichtigste Botschaft in diesem Buch lautet: Die Eltern sind dafür verantwortlich, was zum Essen angeboten wird und die Art und Weise, wie es angeboten wird. Die Kinder sind dafür verantwortlich, wieviel sie essen und ob sie essen wollen. Damit wendet sich die Autorin einerseits gegen Einseitigkeit und Vernachlässigung im angebotenen Speiseplan, andererseits gegen Druck, Zwang und Tricks, mit denen Kinder zum Essen gezwungen werden sollen. Dieser Leitsatz zieht sich mehr oder weniger als roter Faden durch das ganze Buch. Das fängt beim Säugling, Brust- oder Flaschenkind, an, wo die Mutter sich nach den Signalen richten sollte, die vom Kind ausgehen, nicht aber von allgemeinen Vorschriften oder von ihren Vorstellungen. Das gilt — altersgerecht — für Kleinkinder, Vorschulkinder, Schulkinder und Teenager. Das wird mit verschiedenen Anpassungen angewandt auch auf Kinder, die schlecht wachsen, die Gefahr laufen, fett zu werden, bei Essensstörungen und bei Kindern mit besonderen Bedürfnissen, die entwicklungsgestört oder krank sind oder sonst unter Handicaps leiden. Ein Kapitel über Grunddaten, Ernährungsempfehlungen, Lebensmittelvorschläge und die verschiedenen Lebensmittelgruppen beschließt das Buch. 25—30% aller Kinder sollen Eßprobleme haben (meist nach Auffassungen der Eltern), essen zu viel, zu wenig oder das Falsche. Sie haben Schwierigkeiten im Erlernen der Mechanismen im Eßverhalten, zeigen unerfreuliches Verhalten bei Tisch und bizarre Lebensmittelvorlieben. Viele Probleme werden kasuistisch beleuchtet, an typischen Fällen sowohl von Eltern als auch von Kindern häufige Fehler bzw. belastende Situationen dargestellt und praktikable Lösungswege angeboten. Dabei wird in erster Linie empfohlen, das Fehlverhalten der Eltern zu korrigieren. Kinder sind im Prinzip imstande, ihren Lebensmittelverzehr zu regulieren — und das bereits schon im Säuglingsalter. Im allgemeinen reagieren sie auf unbekannte Lebensmittel negativ, akzeptieren sie aber im Laufe der Zeit mit zunehmender Erfahrung und Vertrautheit. Die Eltern können diese Prozesse entweder unterstützen oder aber stören. Wenn Kinder kein Interesse am Essen und an Lebensmitteln zeigen, liegt das Problem nicht darin, daß sie kein Bedürfnis nach essen haben, sondern dann liegen irgendwelche anderen Gründe vor. Das hat vielfach mit negativen Erfahrungen der Kinder mit ihren Eltern zu tun. Ein Kind hat natürliche Signale für Hunger und Sättigung, wenn sie umgestoßen werden, wird das Eßverhalten gestört. Die beste Erziehung vermittelt den Kindern Liebe und Grenzen, das gilt allgemein, das gilt besonders auch im anerzogenen Ernährungsverhalten.

H. HAENEL

Polychlorinated Biphenyls (PCBs): Mammalian and Environmental Toxicology (Environmental Toxin Series 1). Herausgegeben von S. SAFE. 152 Seiten, 33 Abb., 35 Tab. Springer-Verlag, Berlin, Heidelberg, New York, London, Paris, Tokyo 1987. Preis: 98,— DM.

Diese neue Serie (deren Titel etwas irreführend gewählt wurde) beschäftigt sich in ihrem ersten Band mit einer Problemstellung, die sowohl historische als auch aktuelle Bezüge aufweist. Mit wachsendem zeitlichen Abstand vom Zeitpunkt der Erkennung der Gefährdung von Umwelt und Organismen durch PCB's rundet sich das Wissen um ursächliche Zusammenhänge ab und die Durchdringung molekularer Aspekte (dies erfolgt auch in div. Beiträgen) wird möglich. Über PCB's existieren bereits gute Übersichten in der Buch- und Zeitschriftenliteratur. So wird der Leser zu Recht von einem derartigen Band Herausragendes bezüglich Inhalt und Gestaltung erwarten können. Die Beiträge befassen sich mit dem Vorkommen, der Analytik der PCB's, mit ihren biologischen Effekten beim Warmblüter (speziell der Carcinogenität und Mutagenität) und der Biotransformation (einschließlich pharmakokinetischer Modellierung). Hervorzuheben ist ein Kapitel „PCB's und menschliche Gesundheit". Zwischen den einzelnen Kapiteln gibt es Überschneidungen; der Leser erhält an verschiedenen Stellen Übersichten zur Struktur der PCB's usw. Von einer derartigen Monographie hätte sich der Rezensent einen streng systematischen Aufbau der Wissensvermittlung gewünscht, was auch eine erneute Übersichtsarbeit gerechtfertigt hätte. Einige größere Überblicke über analytische Daten sind aus verschiedenen Originalarbeiten übernommen worden. Leider erfolgte dies ohne zusammenfassende Bearbeitung, sondern nur so, daß man im Bedarfsfalle ohnehin auf die Quellen wird zurückgreifen müssen (weil keine exakten Trennbedingungen angegeben worden sind). Literatur wird reichlich, jedoch in der Monographie in uneinheitlicher Form zitiert. Die einzelnen Beiträge sind von den namhaften Autoren in straff gegliederter, übersichtlicher und überwiegend reich illustrierter Form gestaltet. Band 2 wird methodischen Aspekten der Toxizitätsermittlung und dem Cadmium gewidmet sein. Die Publikation erscheint durchaus preiswert.

R. MACHOLZ

Corrections

In the article of A. S. DIMOGLO, M. YU. GORBACHOV, I. B. BERSUKER, A. I. GRENI, L. E. VYSOTSKAYA, O. V. STEPANOVA and E. YU. LUKASH "Structural and electronic origin of meat odour of organic heteroatomic compounds" in issue 5/1988, pp. 461—473, the following errors should be corrected:

1. Pages 462 and 464: In the head of table 1 should be changed
   — twice "see Table 2" in 'see Fig. 1"
   — "Table 3" in "Table 2".
2. Page 465, text line 7: "78 × 12 matrix" should be changed in "77 × 12 matrix".
3. Page 467, text line 1: "Table 4" should be changed in "Table 3".
4. Page 468, text line 6: "The compounds (7)" should be changed in "The compounds (3)".
5. The chemical formula from page 469 is to insert in page 468, text line 19, immediately behind "to a methyl group:".
6. Page 471: The correct structural formula of compound 31 must be:

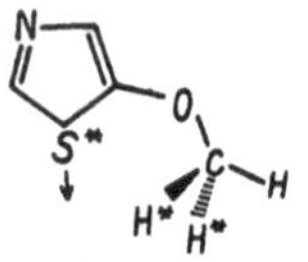

INHALTSVERZEICHNIS

DIE NAHRUNG — FOOD

Volume 32 | 1988 | Number 9

CONTENTS

Die Nahrung — Food is indexed, abstracted or cited in Current Contents/Agriculture, Biology & Environmental Sciences; Science Citation Index; Food Science and Technology Abstracts; Index Medicus; Analytical Abstracts; Chemical Abstracts.

Kolibri 360 GmbH
Ferdinand-Jühlke-Straße 7
99095 Erfurt, Deutschland
produktsicherheit@kolibri360.de